Michelle Foland

Pathophysiology

Definition of Pathophysiology

The term "pathophysiology" comes from the Greek word "pathos," which means "suffering." "physis" means nature, origin; The study of abnormal changes in body functions that are the causes, consequences, or concomitants of disease processes is referred to as "logos," which means "the study of." Changes in the endocrine system, certain neurotransmitters, or inflammatory parameters related to the activity of the immune system are examples of biological processes that are directly related to disease processes of physical, mental, or psychophysiological conditions and disorders that are the focus of pathophysiology studies. As a result, the goal of pathophysiological research is to discover biological mechanisms and markers that can predict and explain disease processes in terms of etiology and pathogenesis. Pathophysiology is officially classified as a branch of physiology.

Understanding SARS-Cov-2's Epidemiology, Pathophysiology, Diagnosis, and Treatment

The coronavirus disease 2019 (COVID-19) exploded onto the global scene in December 2019 with over 20 million cases and 741,808 deaths, affecting over 200 nations. The World Health Organization announced on March 11, 2020, that COVID-19 was a pandemic. The infection is brought about by serious intense respiratory condition Covid 2 (SARS-CoV-2). There is restricted data on Coronavirus, and treatment has up to this point zeroed in on strong consideration and utilization of reused drugs. Droplet spread, or contact between people, is one method by which COVID-19 can be spread. Social distancing, practicing good hygiene, and staying away from crowded areas are some of the recommended preventative measures to cut down on the rate at which the disease spreads. Because the droplets are heavy and can only travel about one meter in the air before quickly settling on fixed surfaces, these measures work. The discovery of therapeutic targets/drugs and vaccines are promising strategies for combating SARS-CoV-2. The epidemiology, pathophysiology, and diagnosis of COVID-19 are summarized in this review. In addition, we discuss the therapeutic management of the disease through the mechanisms of action of approved repurposed drugs.

Introduction

One of the most dangerous pandemics in recent history is COVID-19. More than 740,000 people have died as a result of the pandemic, and more than 20 million cases have been reported since the initial outbreak. The sickness is brought about by SARS-CoV-2, a zoonotic microbe that procured changes as it crossed the species boundary from bat to pangolin empowering it to taint humans.1 SARS-CoV-2 was affirmed as a novel Covid utilizing sub-atomic strategies and at first named 2019 novel Covid (2019-nCoV).2 The illness brought about by this infection was subsequently renamed Coronavirus by the World Wellbeing Association (WHO).3 SARS-CoV-2 is profoundly irresistible and has spread to in excess of 200 nations in all landmasses. As a result, the World Health Organization (WHO) designated the virus as a pandemic threat. The positive sense RNA genome (+ssRNA) of SARS-CoV-2 is approximately 30 kilobases long. Using phylogenetic analysis, it was discovered that the SARS-CoV-2 genome shares 96% sequence similarity with a bat CoV genome.4 The genomes of SARS-CoV-1 and Middle East respiratory syndrome (MERS)-CoV are similarly organized. Due to the widespread distribution of angiotensin converting enzyme-2 (ACE-2), the primary receptor for SARS coronaviruses, in multiple organs, many SARS-CoV-2 deaths have resulted in multiple organ dysfunction syndrome (MSOF) rather than respiratory failure.9,10 ACE-2 is expressed as a cell-surface molecule in the respiratory tract (epithelium, arterial and venous endothelium), the small intestinal epithelium, and arterial smooth muscle It is interesting to note that countries with the highest reported prevalence and mortality rates, such as China, the United States, Spain, Italy, the United Kingdom, Russia, Germany, Brazil, France, Turkey, and Iran, are more concerned with flattening the curve by identifying early cases, isolating them, and developing therapeutic vaccines and drugs. There is insufficient information regarding risk factors for severe outcomes due to the novel nature of this disease. It is still unclear about specific factors like the serial interval, viral lifespan, incubation period, pathogenic mechanisms, clinical features, and the best way to treat the disease. Subsequently, this survey meant to sum up the study of disease transmission and pathophysiology of SARS-CoV-2 as well as the utilization of reused Food and Medication Organization (FDA) supported drugs for treatment. It is important to pay closer attention to this virus's entry into host cells and any potential complications that may follow.

Coronaviruses (CoVs) belong to the family Coronaviridae and the subfamily Othocoronavirinae. There are four genera in the subfamily: alpha, beta, gamma, and delta CoVs.13 While the gamma and delta CoVs only infect birds, the alpha and beta CoVs are capable of infecting mammals, including humans.14 About seven CoVs have been isolated from humans. Human coronavirus 229E (HCoV-229E) and human coronavirus NL63 (HCoV-NL63) are two of these, as are five beta-CoVs: SARS-CoV-1, MERS-CoV, and SARS-CoV-2, human coronavirus OC43 (HCoV-OC43), and human coronavirus HKU1 (HCoV-HKU1). After coming into contact with the respective intermediate hosts (bats), the pathogenic SARS-CoV-1, MERS-CoV, and SARS-CoV-2 cause severe infections in humans. However, it does not appear that HCoV-229E, HCoV-NL63, HCoV-OC43, or HCoV-HKU1 infect humans with severe infections.

CoVs are wrapped infections with +ssRNA genomes. Among RNA viruses, they have the largest genomes (approximately 26–33 kb). The non-segmented genomes of all CoVs are organized in a similar way.15 In general, about two-thirds of the genome is made up of two large, overlapping open reading frames (ORF1a and ORF1b). These ORFs are translated into the polyproteins pp1a and pp1ab, which are then processed to make 16 non-structural proteins (nsp1 to nsp16). The remaining one-third of the genome is because the S protein is involved in virus entry into host cells and binding to receptors, it is regarded as a major therapeutic target. Overview of the SARS-CoV family The SARS-CoVs are a global family of viruses that cause respiratory disease and influenza-like symptoms like fever, muscle pain, sore throat, headache, and cough. The N protein is required for the synthesis of RNA. A pneumonia-like syndrome (MERS) was first discovered in Saudi Arabia and then spread to several countries, where it incurred a mortality rate of approximately 3% to 6%.

In the early 2000s, the outbreak that resulted from the first case of SARS-CoV-1, which was reported in China, resulted in hundreds of deaths and thousands of infected cases.[20] Mara et al [21] saw that the MERS death rate expanded with age and was essentially as high as 43% to 55% in individuals more established than 60 years. SARS-CoV-2 caused an outbreak in China in December 2019 before spreading worldwide. People who have compromised immune systems or underlying conditions like lung disease, diabetes mellitus, and human immunodeficiency virus infection are particularly vulnerable to the disease that results (COVID-19).

SARS-CoV-1

SARS-CoV-1 is a virus that causes a viral respiratory disease and belongs to lineage B of the beta-CoVs. The first human case of SARS-CoV1 infection was found in China in 2002. Within a year, there were approximately 8,422 cases worldwide, affecting 29 countries.[13] Bats are the primary hosts of this virus, with palm civets acting as an intermediate host. Humans contract the disease either through direct contact with intermediate hosts or through the consumption of raw meat, milk, or urine. Human SARS-CoV-1 infections can also spread from person to person through nosocomial transmission. Common symptoms of human SARS-CoV-1 infections include fever, headache, and respiratory complications like pneumonia, dyspnea, and cough.

The length of the SARS-CoV-1 genome is 29,727 nucleotides. ORF1a and ORF1b are located at the genome's fifth end. Several viral proteases and the RNA-dependent RNA polymerase (RdRp) are produced by auto-catalyzing the polyproteins encoded by these ORF. The SARS-CoV receptor is ACE-2, a surface molecule that is found on cells of the respiratory tract, the small intestinal epithelium, and smooth muscle. The remainder of the genome encodes the viral structural proteins (S, E, M, and N) as well as a number of accessory proteins. Alveolar monocytes and macrophages, as well as epithelial cells of the bronchi, trachea, and bronchial serous glands, express ACE-2 in the respiratory tract.

MERS-CoV

MERS-CoV is a virus that causes a viral respiratory disease and belongs to lineage C of the beta-CoVs. In

2012, the first human cases of MERS-CoV infection were reported in Saudi Arabia. The ACE-2 enzyme plays a significant role in protecting against lung failure. After coming into contact with infected camels, cases were then reported in Qatar, Egypt, and the Republic of Korea. Between 2012 and 2018, cases of MERS-CoV were found in about 27 countries.18 MERS-CoV RNA from camels shared more than 99 percent of its genomic sequence with human MERS-CoV.23 Bats are the natural hosts of MERS-CoV , and the Middle East, Spain, and Africa all confirmed a high prevalence of MERS-CoV infections in dromedary camels (intermediate hosts). MERS-CoV contaminations were sent to people following contact with camels tainted with the virus.23

The MERS-CoV genome is around 30,119 nucleotides long and has a 5′ terminal cap structure and a poly (A) tail at the 3′ end. The genome encodes 16 non-primary proteins (nsp1-nsp16) at the 5′ end, four primary proteins (S, E, M, and N) at the 3′ end,24 and five frill proteins in ORF3, ORF4a, ORF4b, ORF5, and ORF8.18 Hazard factors for serious MERS-CoV incorporate age and the presence of fundamental circumstances like diabetes, heftiness, hypertension, constant renal illness, and lung diseases.25

The receptor for MERS-CoV is dipeptidyl peptidase 4 (DPP4 or CD26). DPP4 is a multifunctional cell surface protein and is communicated on the epithelial cells of the respiratory plot, liver, kidney, small digestive tract, and prostate, as well as on initiated white platelets. DPP4 likewise assumes an imperative part in enactment of Lymphocytes and giving co-stimulatory signs to resistant reactions of T cells.11, 18 Subsequently, MERS-CoV causes intense pneumonia and renal brokenness with related clinical side effects, for example, hack, chest torment, sore throat, fever, loose bowels, retching, and stomach torment.

SARS-CoV-2

SARS-CoV-2, a newly discovered coronavirus, has a +ssRNA genome and a spherical morphology when observed under the electron microscope. SARS-CoV-2 encodes a richly glycosylated spike protein responsible for binding to the ACE-2 receptor.28 The virion's shape and the ability of spike proteins to form a crown-like structure gave coronaviruses their name.29, Hemagglutinin, the membrane, the envelope, and the nucleocapsids are additional structural components. The nucleocapsid aids in the packaging of RNA during virion assembly.33, 34 Hemagglutinin enhances the entry and pathogenesis of coronaviruses. Some of the characteristics of SARS-CoV-2 are summarized in Table 1. The membrane exists in greater quantities within the virions than the envelope. Among other functions, the envelope serves to release viral particles from the host cells.32 SARS-CoV-1 shares many of these characteristics with it. The epidemiology and general characteristics of SARS-CoV-1 are covered in greater detail later in the review.

Other important human coronaviruses include two beta-CoVs (HCoV OC43 and HCoV HKU1) and two alpha-CoVs (HCoV 229E and HCoV NL63). Human aminopeptidase N (CD13), a cell surface metalloprotease that is found on kidney, lung, epithelial, and intestinal cells, is the receptor for HCoV229E. ACE-2 is also the HCoVNL63 receptor. In general, molecular detection methods like reverse transcription-polymerase chain reaction (RT-PCR) using RNA extracted from respiratory tract samples as a template are the most common diagnostic tools for human CoVs. The receptor for HCoV OC43 is 9-O-acetylated sialic acid, but there is no receptor for HCoV HKU1. Although several agents against CoVs, such as antibodies, antiviral peptides, and cell or viral protease inhibitors, have been shown to be effective both in vitro and/or in vivo, clinical trial outcomes have not been reported. As a result, clinical treatments for CoVs are still lacking. Other methods include serological tests and viral cultures. Nevertheless, treatment consists of supportive and symptomatic therapy. The most frequently included antiviral agents in combination therapies are interferons, ribavirin, lopinavir/ritonavir, and cyclophilin inhibitors. Type I interferons were reportedly used against MERS-CoV in various cell lines and in rhesus macaques. In cell cultures, interferon-alpha 2b and ribavirin work together to kill SARS-CoV-1 and MERS-CoV.44.

The Study of Disease Transmission of Coronavirus

Coronavirus, the sickness brought about by SARS-CoV-2, is like that brought about by SARS-CoV-1. In December 2019, COVID-19 was first identified in Wuhan, China. Probably during pangolin zoonotic transmission, the virus changed and eventually infected humans. The case casualty rate (CFR) of Coronavirus was assessed at 5.93% (3 June 2020). There were 20,394,078 confirmed cases of SARS-CoV-2 worldwide at the time of writing 741,808 deaths, and over 13,283,665 recovered cases, according to data from Johns Hopkins University.

The SARS-CoV-2 outbreak currently affects 215 nations and territories, including Nigeria, Italy, South Africa, and the United States. Case numbers and mortality rates are high in China, some European nations, and the United States. Worldwide recovery rates are rising, with China reporting higher rates.

The COVID-19 CFR

The CFR is the percentage of deaths among cases that have been confirmed. A CFR of 6.33 percent was estimated for 126,066 to 1,992,189 deaths among confirmed cases on April 14, 2020. This is different from the CFR of 3.70 percent that was calculated on March 15, 2020. However, the CFR may not be accurately determined due to a number of factors. The global CFR and the African CFR were compared. The denominator—the number of confirmed cases—presents a significant obstacle to accurate calculation of the CFR. High CFRs reflect limitations in health care systems, including limited capacity of surveillance systems to trigger a timely response, as well as limited access to health care for the most vulnerable patients (WHO, 2020). Asymptomatic cases of COVID-19, patients with mild symptoms, or individuals who are misdiagnosed may be left out of the denominator, resulting in an underestimation or overestimation of the CFR.

Estimation of the reproductive number of COVID-19 cases Worldwide, more than 20 million cases have been reported to date. It means quite a bit to gauge the regenerative number for this infection to empower exact expectations. Two essential factors, the conceptive proportion (Ro) and the sequential stretch (SI), are crucial for gauge the pace of transmission of this illness.

The degree of COVID-19 contagion or infectiousness is measured by the reproductive ratio (Ro) of COVID-19. Ro is the typical number of people who will be infected by a single infected person. For early COVID-19 outbreaks, Zhang ET al.46 estimated that the median and 95 percent confidence interval (CI) of Ro were approximately 2.28 (2.06–2.52). This indicates that an infected individual can typically spread COVID-19 to two to three other individuals. The serial interval (SI) from the onset of illness in a primary case to the onset of illness in a secondary case is important for understanding the case turnover and transmissibility of COVID-19. Recent studies estimated the average SI for COVID-19 at 3.77 (2.23–4.82) days.49–51 A shorter SI makes COVID-19 harder to contain and more likely to rapidly transmit within populations. Taking the R0 and SI of COVID-19 into consideration, it can be inferred that. Almost certainly, the individual can contaminate around a few different people, making the spread of Coronavirus incredibly fast and perilous. If R0 is less than 1, less than one new infection is caused by each existing infection. The disease will deteriorate and eventually die in this scenario. If Ro is one, one new infection is caused by each existing infection. The population will not experience an epidemic, but the disease will remain stable. If R0 > 1, each current disease causes more than one new contamination. The disease will spread from person to person, eventually resulting in an outbreak. With a R0 greater than 1, COVID-19 was considered an outbreak on January 30, 2020.

Importantly, a disease's R0 value only applies when the entire population is susceptible. This means that no one has ever been infected with the disease or been vaccinated against it, and there is no way to stop it from spreading through drugs or vaccines.

COVID-19 Pathophysiology

There are currently two modes of COVID-19 transmission that are known: the oral-feces route and respiratory droplets. Droplets have the potential to come into contact with a healthy person and infect them within one meter to three to six feet. Sticky droplets can persist for more than 24 hours and remain infectious. The virus can survive in the air for about three hours, which is long enough to allow transmission.

Surfactant production is carried out by type II alveolar pneumocystis, which are infected when SARS-CoV-2 enters the body.57 Alveolar surface tension and collapse pressure are both reduced by surfactant. The virus's spike protein binds to ACE-2 on the pneumocystis, allowing the virion to enter the host cell. The virus takes over the machinery of the host cell (ribosomes) to enable the translation of it's +ssRNA genome into various protein molecules. Within the host cell, the translated polyproteins are further processed into various individual components. Multiple virions are produced through these processes, and when pneumocystis are damaged, they are released. Type II pneumocystis respond to this by releasing specific inflammatory mediators that direct macrophages to secrete tumor necrosis factor-alpha and interleukins 1 and 6 (IL-1 and IL-6) The dilation of the endothelial cells that line blood vessels by these cytokines increases the permeability of the capillaries. Fluids build up in the alveoli as a result, resulting in edema59. The alveoli's collapsing pressure rises in tandem with an increase in surface tension. This process also causes a decrease in gas exchange, which in turn causes hypoxia and dyspnea, or difficulty breathing. A critical condition like acute respiratory distress syndrome (ARDS) can arise as a result of this.

Neutrophils are further stimulated by inflammatory mediators, which trigger the release of proteases and reactive oxygen species. Alveoli of type 1 and 2 suffer damage as a result of this process, which results in alveolar consolidation and collapse. The hypothalamus is instructed to release prostaglandins, triggering a fever, and high levels of IL-1 and IL-6 travel through the blood to the central nervous system. Systemic inflammatory respiratory syndrome is caused by severe lung inflammation. Capillary permeability can increase with progression. Multiple system organ failure (MSOF) can result from a series of processes that include hypotension and decreased perfusion of multiple organs as the overall blood volume decreases. The kidney accumulates elevated levels of blood urea, nitrogen, and creatinine during MSOF. Aspartate transaminase, alanine transaminase, bilirubin, C - reactive protein [CRP], fibrinogen, and interleukin-6 (IL-6) are inflammatory and acute phase response biomolecules released by the liver that can be used as biomarkers for COVID-19 patients.

Transmission of SARS-Cov-2 through the Eyes

Several groups continue to investigate the mechanism by which SARS-CoV-2 is transmitted through the eyes. Because health care providers, including a physician at Perking University, may have contracted the virus while treating patients without wearing eye protection, investigations were required.61 Some researchers have asserted that avoiding touching the eyes, nose, or mouth with hands that have not been washed or sterilized can reduce COVID-19 transmission. SARS-CoV-2 upper respiratory tract infections can cause ocular symptoms like viral conjunctivitis, which was confirmed in 9 of 1,099 patients in China.64 Other research also found that 1 of 30 patients hospitalized with COVID-19 was diagnosed with conjunctivitis.65 In a study that was carried out by the American Optometric Association, COVID-19 was linked to ocular signs and symptoms like photophobia, irritation, conjunctival infection, and ocular discharge

SARS-CoV-2's clinical manifestations are ambiguous and fluctuate frequently. COVID-19 symptoms A few contaminations are asymptomatic. Respiratory distress syndrome, pneumonia of varying degrees of severity67, and occasionally death are all possible signs. Fever, fatigue, a dry, persistent cough, and shortness of breath are the most common symptoms of COVID-19, according to the World Health Organization (WHO).68,69 Other symptoms include runny nose, sore throat, nasal congestion, aches and pains, diarrhea, and a loss of sense of smell and taste.70 Patients who are critically ill with COVID-19 may also present with increased venous thromboembolism, including thrombocytopenia, elevated D-dimer, prolonged prothrombin time, and disseminated intravascular coagulation (DIC). The least common symptoms include nausea or vomiting, coughing up blood or bloody mucus, and viral conjunctivitis, which causes red eyes, watery discharge from the eyes, swollen eyelids, and a systemic inflammatory response and an imbalance in the homeostasis mechanisms of pro- and anticoagulants are linked to these abnormalities in coagulation and raise mortality risk74. Some of these clinical characteristics are also seen in cases of DIC in septic patients. Due to the fact that their levels are higher than the standards for sepsis, COVID-19 patients exhibit very distinct characteristics.

SARS-CoV-2 diagnosis, prognosis, treatment, and management SARS-CoV-2 causes a variety of complications, including pneumonia, fever, and decreased organ perfusion that leads to MSOF. The primary diagnostic tests for SARS-CoV-2 that use nasal swabs, aspirate, sputum, or blood as samples are quantitative polymerase chain reaction-based (qPCR) methods77. Because COVID-19's early symptoms are similar to those of influenza, a nasopharyngeal swab test is the first step in distinguishing it from influenza and pneumonia. The newly approved nucleic acid test, which is carried out based on the principle of fluorescence PCR, is another diagnostic method.81 The primary objective of SARS-CoV-2 diagnosis is to accurately detect the virus and to minimize further transmissions by promptly isolating and treating infected patients. These methods have some limitations due to their time consumption and variable sensitivity (30%–80%).78–80 Clinical manifestations serve as the basis for the use of additional tests that are not specific to SARS-CoV-2. These incorporate blood tests, for example, complete blood count, far reaching metabolic boards, essential metabolic boards, and evaluation of liver/kidney markers and procalcitonin levels (for bacterial contaminations). CRP, erythrocyte sedimentation rate, IL-6, lactate dehydrogenase, D-dimer, ferritin, troponin, and creatine kinase-MB are other inflammatory markers that can be evaluated. Typically, computed tomography scans are used for imaging investigations: In cases of severe and progressive disease, these frequently exhibit glass opacities, consolidation areas, and paving patterns. Ground glass opacities can likewise be seen on chest X-beam. At last, ultrasound can show B-lines, pleural line thickening, and lung solidification. Assessment can also be done with air bronchograms. These non-specific tests are useful for determining a patient's health status.

Coronavirus patients with extreme ARDS might actually give pneumonia. Pneumonia can be very bad, and it can cause ARDS and MSOF. It is in this manner basic to precisely ventilate the lungs to keep away from ARDS and MSOF.

Prognosis for SARS-COV-2 Despite the fact that the risk factors for COVID-19 are still unknown, some risk factors significantly increase mortality risk, particularly in patients with underlying conditions.6,35,40,82 Some medical disorders are linked to an increased mortality risk in COVID-19 patients. These include cardiovascular diseases (mortality risk of 10.6 percent), 41 lung diseases (mortality risk of 7.3 percent), type 1 and type 2 diabetes (mortality risk of 6.3 percent), and immunosuppression (for example, cancer patients; mortality risk (5.6%), age, and ages 83–86.87 COVID-19 mortality rates rise with age, and are particularly high in people over 60. Raised provocative markers in light of tissue harm (raised degrees of D-dimer, ferritin, creatine kinase-MB, and troponin) have been related with higher death rates.

Self-quarantine for at least 14 days is the first line of treatment for patients who present with COVID-19 symptoms (fever, dry cough, and shortness of breath). The progression of symptoms like an elevated temperature (>40°C), significant difficulty breathing or shortness of breath, mouth breaks, persistent coughing, and dehydration is monitored in each case. Consult a doctor for confirmation of the diagnosis and to prevent the virus from spreading further if symptoms do not significantly improve. Supportive care is currently the most common type of treatment. There has been a connection between COVID-19 and ARDS, despite the limited information available. For patients with high fevers that might actually prompt drying out, intravenous liquids, for example, typical saline or lactated Ringer's liquid can be managed sparingly to forestall lung over-burden. Antipyretic medications like acetaminophen or paracetamol can be given to lower the temperature. Medications, for example, remdesivir, chloroquine, ritonavir, tocilizumab, corticosteroids have been reused for the treatment of Coronavirus in spite of the fact that their clinical adequacy has not yet been confirmed.[88-93] Sadly, the utilization of chloroquine and subordinates like hydroxychloroquine, alone or in mix with different medications, brought about cardiovascular poisonousness. The World Health Organization (WHO) recently halted research into these drugs.

Select Repurposed Drugs' Mechanisms of Action for COVID-19 Treatment

The identification of potential targets may lead to COVID-19-specific treatments. Inhibition of SARS-CoV-2 entry, disruption of SARS-CoV-2 +ssRNA synthesis following entry, suppression of the inflammatory response, and disruption of SARS-CoV-2 translation are all approaches to the development of anti-SARS-CoV-2 drugs.

Remdesivir, a novel antiviral drug and nucleotide analog used to treat Ebola virus infection, is currently in clinical development. Remdesivir can inhibit the entry of COVID-19 into the endosome after binding to ACE-2 receptors, preventing the release of +ssRNA for translation. Studies also showed that hydroxychloroquine, an analog of chloroquine, was more potent and could be used in place of chloro The drug is thought to work at the post-viral entry stage, inhibiting the RdRp and preventing the synthesis of the viral +ssRNA. Clinical trials for this drug are currently in phase 2. Ritonavir, a protein inhibitor, has also been suggested as a treatment for COVID-19. By inhibiting the conversion of polyproteins into the mature components (spike proteins, nucleocapsids) required by the virus for its multiplication, this medication affects the protease enzymes (proteinases). Due to its capacity to inhibit inflammatory responses and block IL-6, tocilizumab, another immunosuppressive medication, has also been repurposed for COVID-19. By inhibiting phospholipases like phospholipase A2, corticosteroids can also reduce inflammation and suppress the excessive production of prostaglandins

The human innate immune system does not appear to be familiar with SARS-CoV-2. The development of vaccines for prevention is no longer a matter of debate but rather a necessity in light of its emergence and global spread via human-to-human transmission. There are a number of vaccine platforms in development, some of which have entered clinical trials. However, manufacturing and FDA approval may take 12 to 18 months[98]. Two classes of molecules—protein biogenesis inhibitors and ligands of the Sigma1 and Sigma2 receptors—have been identified as effective inhibitors of viral infectivity in studies of the antiviral activity of host-directed drugs and compounds. The ligands haloperidol, PB28, PD-

144418, and hydroxychloroquine are currently undergoing clinical trials in COVID-19 patients. These molecules exert their antiviral effects during viral replication by inhibiting nucleoprotein expression after viral entry has occurred. Molecules that target the Sigma1 and Sigma2 receptors perturb the virus through a variety of mechanisms from translation inhibitors, possibly including modulation of cellular stress responses.99. A recent study by Gordon et al. identified 332 high-confidence SARS-CoV-2-human protein interactions connected to multiple biological processes, including protein trafficking, translation, transcription, and ubiquitination regulation.102 The study identified 69 ligands, including drugs that have been approved by the FDA, compounds in clinical trials, and preclinical compounds, that may theoretically have therapeutic effects as host-directed interventions against COVID-19. Off-target effects on the human Ether-à-go- There are currently no antiviral medications or vaccines against SARS-CoV-2 that have been shown to be effective in clinical settings. The lack of information about the infection's molecular details may have contributed to the absence of such agents. Understanding how the virus interacts with the host during infection is essential for the development of therapeutic interventions against COVID-19.

The functional receptor for SARS-CoV-2 has been identified as ACE-2, making it a potential target for COVID-19 treatment. It is a type-II transmembrane metallocarboxypeptidase with its enzymatically active domain exposed at the cell surface.104 ACE-2 is a key player in the renin-angiotensin system (RAS) and a target for treatment of hypertension.105 ACE-2 catalyzes the cleavage of angiotensin II into angiotensin 1–7, a vasodilator, Studies have shown that ACE inhibitors and angiotensin II receptor blockers can be used to up-regulate the expression and activity of ACE-2 in hypertensive patients.109,110 Recent studies have shown that the expression of human ACE-2 is associated with SARSCoV infection and that genetic variations of this receptor may contribute to susceptibility and/or resistance against infection.111 For example, a single-cell RNA sequencing analysis of ACE-2 revealed that type II alveolar cells had higher When compared to the six female samples, ACE-2 expression was higher in the two male samples.

Variation in ACE-2 expression in COVID-19 patients is likely to affect susceptibility, symptoms, and intervention outcomes following SARS-CoV-2 infection, as the only Asian male in the study had higher ACE-2 expression than Caucasian and black Americans.59 This may explain why the four German cases had mild clinical symptoms but did not have a severe illness.112

Precautions against COVID-19

The current rate of spread of COVID-19 is approximately 5.3 percent, but this number could rise if preventative measures are not taken. Worldwide counteraction of the spread of Coronavirus is hence a critical and pressing objective. It is of the utmost importance to identify and isolate people who have COVID-19 in order to stop the disease from spreading further. Self-quarantine, isolation of infected individuals, social isolation, good personal hygiene (frequent hand washing with soap and water or alcohol-based sanitizers and avoiding touching the eyes, nose, and mouth), and the use of personal protective equipment are examples of measures to prevent spread. Soap can assemble into bubble-like structures known as micelles that trap viral matter and other biomaterials.114 Surfactants in soap lather have their hydrophilic parts pointing outwards and interacting with solvent, while their hydrophobic heads pointing inwards. These classes of compounds have the ability to neutralize microbes such as SARS CoV-2.113 Surfactants in soap can disrupt and sequester viruses and other contaminants, whereas sanitizers and disinfectants are designed to kill SARS-CoV-2. This opens the outer membrane of the coronavirus and encapsulates viral molecules within micelles. This makes insoluble viral molecules easily soluble in water and effectively removes them from hands, surfaces, or other areas after approximately 20 seconds.

In conclusion, the SARS-CoV-2 outbreak now poses a global threat. However, there is still a lack of information regarding this virus. There is inconsistency in the information that is available, and data are updated frequently, which may contribute to differences in study results. Well-annotated data from clinical patients and subclinical subjects in normal populations could help to better understand the pandemic for more consistent and accurate results.

The data gave in this survey depends on information gave by the Middle to Frameworks Science and Designing (CSSE) at Johns Hopkins College during explicit date ranges. The prevalence of SARS-CoV-2, its pathophysiology, diagnosis, and potential treatment are all summarized here. To address the current difficulties in the search for adequate vaccines, diagnostics, and treatments, research efforts are intensifying. Until relevant targets and therapies are discovered, clinical studies into the genetic variation of receptors like ACE-2 across populations and tissues will continue to be an active area of research. While the advancement of satisfactory medicines and antibodies for Coronavirus is in progress, it is prudent that great cleanliness works on including washing of hands and social separating ought to be drilled, and government direction/rules ought to be observed. The disease's spread will be slowed down as a result of this. We anticipate that the insights gleaned from this review will make it possible for researchers to assist patients in developing more accommodating lifestyles and boost the effectiveness of healthcare provider.

The Importance Of This Abstract Is: Coronavirus Disease 2019 (COVID-19): Pathophysiology, Transmission, Diagnosis, and Treatment

Due to the novel severe acute respiratory syndrome coronavirus 2 (SARS-CoV-2), the coronavirus disease 2019 (COVID-19) pandemic has resulted in a sudden and significant increase in pneumonia with multiorgan disease hospitalizations all over the world. This survey examines current proof with respect to the pathophysiology, transmission, determination, and the executives of Coronavirus.

Observations: SARS-CoV-2 is spread essentially by means of respiratory drops during close eye to eye contact. Carriers who are asymptomatic, presymptomatic, or both can spread an infection. 97.5 percent of people who develop symptoms do so within 11.5 days, and the average time between exposure and onset of symptoms is 5 days. Fever, shortness of breath, and a dry cough are the most typical symptoms. Nonspecific radiographic and laboratory abnormalities include lymphopenia and elevated lactate dehydrogenase. Reverse transcription polymerase chain reaction testing is used to identify SARS-CoV-2, though up to 67% of patients may receive false-negative results; however, this is contingent on the timing and quality of the tests. Asymptomatic carriers and fulminant disease characterized by sepsis and acute respiratory failure are examples of COVID-19 manifestations. Approximately 5% and 20% of COVID-19 patients who are admitted to a hospital experience severe symptoms that necessitate intensive care. More than 75% of COVID-19 patients in hospitals need more oxygen. Best practices for supportive management of acute hypoxic respiratory failure are included in COVID-19 treatment. Dexamethasone treatment appears to have a lower 28-day mortality rate in patients who require supplemental oxygen than usual care (21.6 percent vs. 24.6%; age-adjusted rate ratio, 0.83 [95% CI, 0.74-0.92]), and that remdesivir reduces recovery time from 15 to 11 days (hospital discharge or no need for supplemental oxygen). Convalescent plasma did not speed up recovery in 103 COVID-19 patients in a randomized study. Immune modulators, anticoagulants, and antiviral therapies are the subjects of ongoing trials. In the United States, the case-fatality rate for COVID-19 varies significantly by age, from 0.3 deaths per 1000 cases among patients aged 5 to 17 to 304.9 deaths per 1000 cases among patients 85 and older. The case fatality rate for patients admitted to the intensive care unit is up to 40%. At least 120 vaccines against SARS-CoV-2 are in development. Face masks, social distance, and contact tracing are the primary strategies for reducing spread until an effective vaccine is developed. Hyperimmune globulin and monoclonal antibodies are two potential additional methods of prevention.

Relevance and findings: As of July 1, 2020, in excess of 10 million individuals overall had been tainted with SARS-CoV-2. There are still many unknowns regarding infection, transmission, and treatment. Propels in counteraction and successful administration of Coronavirus will require fundamental and clinical examination and general wellbeing and clinical mediations.

Pathophysiology of Type 2 Diabetes Mellitus

Type 2 Diabetes Mellitus (T2DM), perhaps of the most well-known metabolic problem, is brought about by a mix of two essential elements: the inability of insulin-sensitive tissues to respond appropriately to insulin and defective insulin secretion by pancreatic cells. The molecular mechanisms involved in insulin synthesis, release, and detection are tightly regulated because insulin release and activity are necessary for glucose homeostasis. Surrenders in any of the components engaged with these cycles can prompt a metabolic lopsidedness liable for the improvement of the illness. The key features of type 2 diabetes and the molecular mechanisms and pathways that are thought to play a role in insulin metabolism and lead to insulin resistance and T2DM are the subject of this review. For that reason, we sum up the information got together up to this point, zeroing in particularly on insulin blend, insulin discharge, insulin detecting and on the downstream consequences for individual insulin-delicate organs. The pathological conditions that exacerbate T2DM are also discussed, including metabolic memory, gut dysbiosis, and nutritional factors. We also discuss some of the molecular mechanisms that link T2DM and insulin resistance (IR), as well as cardiovascular risk, which is one of the most significant T2DM complications. This is because T2DM is linked to the acceleration of the development of atherosclerosis.

Introduction Type 2 Diabetes Mellitus (T2DM) is one of the most prevalent metabolic disorders in the world. It is primarily brought about by a combination of two primary factors: the inability of insulin-sensitive tissues to respond to insulin and defective insulin secretion by pancreatic cells. The metabolic demand must be precisely met by insulin release and action; subsequently, the atomic components engaged with the combination and arrival of insulin, as well as the insulin reaction in tissues should be firmly directed. As a result, the pathogenesis of T2DM can be caused by a metabolic imbalance caused by flaws in any of the involved mechanisms.

The molecular mechanisms and pathways involved in insulin metabolism, as well as the connections between T2DM and cardiovascular pathophysiology, are all examined in this review. Global T2DM trends and the roles of major risk factors, particularly obesity, lifestyle factors, genetic predispositions, gut dysbiosis, epigenetics, and mitochondrial deregulation, are discussed in this review. We draw attention to the physiological and molecular mechanisms that cause T2DM and the complications it causes.

Diabetes Mellitus Type 2: Background and epidemiology According to the World Health Organization (WHO), diabetes mellitus is a metabolic, chronic disease characterized by high blood glucose levels that eventually cause damage to the heart, vasculature, eyes, kidneys, and nerves. More than 90% of diabetes mellitus cases are T2DM, a condition set apart by insufficient insulin discharge by pancreatic islet β-cells, tissue insulin obstruction (IR) and a lacking compensatory insulin secretory reaction. As the disease progresses, insulin secretion becomes unable to regulate glucose homeostasis, resulting in hyperglycemia. Obesity or a higher body fat percentage, primarily in the abdominal area, are the main characteristics of T2DM patients. Adipose tissue promotes insulin resistance (IR) in this condition through a variety of inflammatory mechanisms, such as increased release of free fatty acids (FFA) and regulation of adipokines. The global rise in obesity, sedentary lifestyles, high-calorie diets, and population aging, which has quadrupled the incidence and prevalence of T2DM, are the primary drivers of the T2DM epidemic.

The pancreas (cells and -cells), liver, skeletal muscle, kidneys, brain, small intestine, and adipose tissue are all involved in the development of T2DM. Developing information recommend a job for adipokine dysregulation, irritation, and irregularities in stomach microbiota, safe dysregulation, and irritation have arisen as significant pathophysiological factors.

Data from epidemiology reveal alarming levels that indicate a bleak outlook for T2DM's future. The International Diabetes Federation (IDF) estimates that diabetes was the cause of 4.2 million deaths in 2019. Additionally, diabetes affected 463 million adults between the ages of 20 and 79, a number that is expected to rise to 700 million by 2045. In 2019, at least 720 billion USD in health care costs were attributed to diabetes. Due to the fact that one in three diabetics, or 232 million people, were not diagnosed, the true burden of T2DM is probably underrepresented. The best number of individuals experiencing diabetes are matured somewhere in the range of 40 and 59 years of age. T2DM incidence and prevalence vary by region, with more than 80% of patients living in low- to middle-income countries, making effective treatment even more difficult. Cardiovascular disease (CVD) is the leading cause of T2DM-related morbidity and mortality, with a 15% increased risk of all-cause mortality compared to those without diabetes. The relationship of diabetes with expanded chance of coronary illness (risk proportion [HR] 2.00; Ischaemic stroke (HR 2.27; 95 percent CI 1.83–2.19), 1.95–2.65), in addition to other deaths caused by vascular disease (HR 1.73; A meta-analysis found that 1.51–1.98)

T2DM's epidemiology is influenced by both genetics and the environment. After being exposed to an environment that encourages sedentary behavior and high calorie intake, genetic factors take effect. Genome-wide association studies have identified common glycemic genetic variants for T2DM, but these only account for 10% of total trait variance, indicating that rare variants are important. Different ethnic groups may have different specific phenotypes that make them more likely to have clusters of cardiovascular disease risk factors like high blood pressure, insulin resistance, and dyslipidemia.

3. Pathophysiology and risk factors for type 2 diabetes include a complicated combination of genetic, metabolic, and environmental factors that interact with one another to increase the risk of the disease. Although non-modifiable risk factors (ethnicity and family history/genetic predisposition) have a strong genetic basis for individual T2DM predisposition, epidemiological studies suggest that improving the main modifiable risk factors (obesity, low physical activity, and unhealthy diet) can prevent many cases.

Ethnicity and Family History/Genetic Predisposition Globally, the incidence and prevalence of type 2 diabetes vary greatly based on ethnicity and geographic location, with Native Americans, Japanese, and Hispanics at greatest risk. Asians have been shown to have higher incidence rates than White Americans and White people in the UK, where

Black people have the highest risk. Although no conclusive cause has been identified, direct genetic propensity or gene-environment interactions, modern lifestyle factors (which encourage obesity), and socioeconomic factors have been proposed as contributing factors.

The risk of developing T2DM is significantly influenced by genetic predisposition. Numerous T2DM genome-wide association studies conducted over the past ten years have demonstrated the complex polygenic nature of T2DM, with the majority of these loci increasing T2DM risk through primary effects on insulin secretion and a minority reducing insulin action. Dimas and co. gathered these variations based on their possible transitional components in T2DM pathophysiology, with four variations fitting an unmistakable IR design; two decreasing insulin emission with fasting hyperglycemia; nine reducing insulin secretion when fasting glycemia is normal; and one that changes how insulin is processed. These data indicate that the genetic architecture of type 2 diabetes is highly polygenic, and additional association studies are required to locate the majority of T2DM loci.

According to observational studies and clinical trials, interactions between susceptibility loci and environmental factors may account for the absence of T2DM heritability. As a result, the impact of a particular genetic variant can be modulated by the environmental factors (and vice versa).

Obesity (body-mass index [BMI] 30 kg/m2) is the most significant risk factor for type 2 diabetes (T2DM) and is linked to metabolic abnormalities that lead to insulin resistance (IR). BMI and the age at diagnosis of T2DM have an inverse linear relationship. It is still unclear how obesity causes T2DM and insulin resistance exactly; this pathological process, which involves both cell-autonomous mechanisms and inter-organ communications, has been shown to be influenced by a variety of factors.

According to the Women's Health Study and the Kuipio Ischemic Heart Disease Risk Factor Study, a sedentary lifestyle is another risk factor for T2DM. Both studies found that participants who walked 2–3 hours a week or at least 40 minutes a week had a 34% and 56% lower risk of developing T2DM, respectively. Physical activity has three main effects on the delay of T2DM onset. First, when skeletal muscle cells contract, more blood flows into the muscle, increasing plasma glucose uptake. Second, active work diminishes the infamous intra-stomach fat, which is a realized gamble factor that advances IR. Finally, it has been demonstrated that moderate exercise can increase glucose uptake by 40%. In addition to enhancing glucose uptake and insulin sensitivity, physical activity has the potential to ameliorate or even reverse T2DM-predisposing factors like inflammation and oxidative stress.

Pathophysiology In terms of the disease's pathophysiology, an abnormally high blood glucose level is caused by a malfunction in the feedback loops between insulin action and insulin secretion. The body's capacity to maintain physiological glucose levels is limited when -cell dysfunction results in reduced insulin secretion. On the other hand, IR causes the liver to produce more glucose and the muscle, liver, and adipose tissue to take in less glucose. Cell dysfunction is typically more severe than IR, even if both processes occur early in the pathogenesis and contribute to the development of the disease. Hyperglycemia, on the other hand, is exacerbated when both IR and -cell dysfunction are present, resulting in the progression of T2DM].

4. Pathophysiology and the underlying mechanisms of type 2 diabetes Production of Insulin: T2DM's Physiological and Dysfunctional Mechanisms -Cell Physiology

To maintain proper cell function, cellular integrity must be maintained, and the physiologic mechanisms and pathways must be tightly regulated.-cells are in charge of making insulin, which is made from pre-proinsulin. Proinsulin is produced when pre-proinsulin undergoes a conformational change during maturation with the assistance of several proteins in the endoplasmic reticulum (ER). After that, proinsulin is moved from the ER to the Golgi apparatus (GA), where it is broken down into insulin and C-peptide in immature secretory vesicles.

Insulin is stored in granules until it is released once it has matured. Insulin discharge is essentially set off by a reaction to high glucose fixations. Amino acids, fatty acids, and hormones are just a few of the other things that can trigger insulin release. The glucose transporter 2 (GLUT2), a solute carrier protein that also serves as a glucose sensor for -cells, is the primary pathway by which -cells absorb glucose when circulating glucose levels rise. When glucose enters the cell, glucose catabolism is started, which raises the intracellular ATP/ADP ratio and causes the plasma membrane's ATP-dependent potassium channels to close. Ca2+ can enter the cell as a result of membrane depolarization and the opening of voltage-dependent Ca2+ channels. Ca2+ signals can be amplified by the RY receptors (RYR) and may play important roles in stimulus-insulin secretion coupling by virtue of their strategic locations within the cell and their ability to mediate Ca2+ induced Ca2+ release (CICR). Additionally, the rise in the intracellular Ca2+ concentration causes the priming and fusion of the secretory insulin-containing granules to the plasma membrane, which results in insulin exocytosis. RYR is involved in the amplification of insulin secretion and amplifies Ca2+ signals when the channel is sensitized by messenger molecules produced during nutrient metabolism or ligand binding.

In any case, other cell signs can likewise help or improve insulin discharge from β-cells. Among them, cAMP may be the main courier potentiating insulin discharge. There is mounting evidence that cAMP increases intracellular Ca2+ concentrations by depleting intracellular Ca2+ reservoirs, thereby triggering insulin-containing secretory vesicle mobilization. Extracellular ATP is another important regulator of -cell function, according to compelling evidence. It is well known that when glucose is applied, -cells release ATP through the exocytosis of insulin granules. Ca2+ mobilization and insulin exocytosis regulation are both regulated and stimulated by purinergic signaling via P2Y and P2X purinergic receptors, independently of glucose. P2X-type receptors are ATP-activated ligand-gated ion channels that are not selective for cations, whereas P2Y purinoreceptors have been reported to be coupled to G-proteins. In the case of P2Y receptors, it has been hypothesized that insulin release may be mediated by intracellular Ca2+ mobilization in response to the formation of inositol-1,4,5-trisphosphate (IP3), which causes the release of Ca2+ from ER stores and amplifies the signal that initiates exocytosis.

Mechanisms That Underlie Cell Dysfunction

Traditionally, cell death has been linked to cell dysfunction. However, the dysfunction of -cells in T2DM may be caused by a more intricate network of interactions between the environment and various cell biology-related molecular pathways, according to recent evidence. Hyperglycemia and hyperlipidemia are common in an excessive nutritional state, similar to obesity, favoring IR and chronic inflammation. Due to differences in their genetic susceptibility, -cells are exposed to toxic pressures like inflammation, inflammatory stress, ER stress, metabolic/oxidative stress, and amyloid stress under these conditions, which have the potential to ultimately result in the loss of islet integrity.

Hyperglycemia and an excess of FFAs cause -cell dysfunction by activating the apoptotic unfolded protein response (UPR) pathways and causing ER stress. In fact, obesity-related lipotoxicity, glucotoxicity, and glucolipotoxicity cause -cell damage through metabolic and oxidative stress. Several mechanisms, including inhibition of the sarco/endoplasmic reticulum Ca2+ ATPase (SERCA) that is responsible for ER Ca2+ mobilization, can activate the UPR pathway in response to stress caused by high levels of saturated FFAs.

IP3 Receptor Activation or Direct ER Homeostasis Disruption

The accumulation of misfolded insulin and islet amyloid polypeptides (IAAP) as well as an increase in the production of oxidative protein folding-mediated reactive oxygen species (ROS) are both consequences of sustained high glucose levels in -cells. Proapoptotic signals are favored, proinsulin mRNA degradation is induced, and interleukin (IL)-1 is released, which recruits macrophages and increases local islet inflammation.

To precisely meet metabolic demand, insulin secretion must be precisely controlled, as previously mentioned. As a result, in order for -cells to respond to metabolic demands, islet integrity must be preserved. The above mechanism can ultimately disrupt islet integrity and organization under pathogenic conditions, preventing optimal cell-to-cell communication within pancreatic islets, contributing to poor insulin and glucagon release regulation, and ultimately escalating hyperglycemia. Insulin secretory dysfunction, which is the primary cause of -cell failure and the foundation of T2DM, can be caused by defects in the synthesis of any insulin precursors or insulin itself, as well as by disruptions in the secretion mechanism. For instance, the downstream signaling pathway would be impacted by decreased expression of the GLUT2 glucose transporter. Failure in the folding of proinsulin is another finding that is frequently associated with diabetes and insufficient insulin production.

Nutritional Factors

The high-caloric Western diet raises blood glucose and circulating very-low-density lipoproteins (VLDLs), chylomicrons (CMs), and their remnants (CMRs), which are rich in triglycerides (TG). Pathological Conditions Perpetuating T2DM This leads to an abnormal production of inflammatory molecules and a rise in the concentration of reactive oxygen species

(ROS). After a substantial meal, a synergistic interaction between the two processes occurs, amplifying negative postprandial effects due to inflammation's acknowledged role as an inducer of oxidative stress. The pathogenesis of T2DM and IR is significantly influenced by the persistent and significant rise in steady-state ROS levels. As a result, mitochondrial dysfunction, ER stress, the activation of NADPH oxidase (NOX), and the production of superoxide (O2) are all consequences of a pro-oxidant environment. The five major pathways that are involved in the pathogenesis of diabetes complications are activated by the increase in O2 production: enhancement of the polyol pathway, expansion of the production of advanced glycation end products (AGEs), expansion of the expression of the AGEs receptor and its activating ligands, expansion of protein kinase C (PKC) isoforms, and expansion of the hexosamine pathway's overactivity. In response to ischemia, increased intracellular ROS activates a number of proinflammatory pathways, causes long-lasting epigenetic changes, and drives persistent expression of proinflammatory genes even after glycemia is normalized through these pathways.

In addition, two distinct mechanisms contribute to mitochondrial dysfunction when blood levels of FFAs are elevated: 1) FFA digestion side-effects upset the electron stream all through the mitochondrial respiratory chain and (2) through the fuse of FFAs into the mitochondrial layers, hence probable inclining toward electron spillage.

Physical Activity There is a link between obesity and T2DM and increased markers of chronic low-grade systemic inflammation, as well as decreased physical activity and exercise training and increased sedentary behaviors. In this condition, proinflammatory molecules like interleukin 6 (IL-6), C-reactive protein (CRP), tumor necrosis factor-alpha (TNF-), or IL-1 induce an inflammatory state called metabolic inflammation within specific tissues. In point of fact, IL-1 plays a role in the autoimmune response that occurs in the pancreas to -cells, which results in the inhibition of -cell function and the activation of the nuclear factor kappa-light-chain-enhancer of activated B cells (NF-B) transcription factor. This results in the inhibition of -cell function and the promotion of apoptosis. Preclinical animal data confirming that deletion of the macromolecular complex NLRP3 inflammasome, which is responsible for the production of IL-1 and IL-18, resulted in improved insulin sensitivity supports the idea that inflammation resolution could prevent the development of T2DM in obesity and prediabetes.

Intentional weight loss is still the most important treatment for improving insulin sensitivity and, in some cases, preventing T2DM in obese and pre-diabetic people. The production of anti-inflammatory cytokines like IL-1 Receptor antagonist (IL-1Ra) and soluble TNF receptor (s-TNF-R), which are antagonists of IL-1 and TNF-, respectively, is boosted by regular exercise and increased physical activity. Leptin, a molecule associated with CRP, and circulating levels of IL-6, IL-18, and CRP are also lower in people who engage in more physical activity. The synthesis of antioxidants like glutathione (GSH), a major non-enzymatic antioxidant, and other antioxidant enzymes, which result in a long-term reduction in free radical levels, can improve T2DM-induced oxidative stress.

Finally, in response to exercise, skeletal muscle and adipose tissue secrete irisin, a myokine that is exercise-regulated and improves glucose tolerance. Irisin levels in the blood of T2DM patients were found to be lower than those of control subjects. Additionally, serum irisin levels in diabetics with CVD were significantly lower than those in non-CVD patients. Low degrees of serum irisin have been related with 1.6 times expanded hazard of CVD occurrence in T2DM patients.

Dysbiosis of the gut

The gut microbiota is made up of numerous microbial species that have an effect on human physiology and take part in various biological processes. They are able to control the inflammatory response and immune system, maintain the integrity of the gut barrier, regulate human metabolism, and participate in the synthesis of metabolites. Numerous metabolites that contribute to physiology in healthy individuals are produced by resident microorganisms in the gut. Nonetheless, changes because of both acquired and gained factors like age, sustenance, way of life, hereditary inclination, or basic illnesses can influence the stomach microbiota created metabolite extent prompting metabolic aggravations that can come full circle in sickness. Recent studies indicate that dysbiosis can promote IR and T2DM, and a better understanding of the gut microbiota has demonstrated its significant role in diabetes development. In models of mice, a diet high in fat has the potential to triple the amount of lipopolysaccharide produced by Gram-negative bacteria, which contributes to insulin resistance and low-grade inflammation. Short-chain fatty acid synthesis, which promotes gut barrier integrity, pancreatic -cell proliferation, and insulin biosynthesis can also be reduced by intestinal dysbiosis. In addition, dysbiosis can impair the production of other metabolites like branched amino acids and trimethylamine, which can lead to the development of T2DM. The field of understanding the clinical implications of the gut microbiome is still in its infancy, and more research is needed to better understand the link between T2DM and the gut microbiota.

Metabolic Memory

The persistence of diabetic complications even when glycemic control is maintained is referred to as metabolic memory. This idea emerged from the findings of numerous large-scale clinical trials, which demonstrated that even when glycemic control is restored through pharmaceutical intervention, diabetes complications persist and progress after the onset of the disease. Among them, the UKPDS post-preliminary review and Steno-2 preliminary showed that explicitly early glycemic mediations forestall diabetic confusion and has an obvious lessening in CVD endpoints in patients that got either standard or concentrated treatment observing their finding. Later, animal diabetes models and in vitro cell cultures demonstrated that the initial hyperglycemic period causes target organs and cells to have permanent abnormalities (such as abnormal gene expression). Metabolic memory includes four instruments: epigenetics, oxidative pressure, non-enzymatic glycation of proteins and constant aggravation.

Epigenetics can control gene expression and determine which proteins are transcribed. It involves genetic modulation by factors other than an individual's DNA sequence. There are various mechanisms for epigenetic regulation: covalent modifications of histone proteins, direct methylation of cytosine or adenine residues, higher-order chromatin structure, and non-coding RNAs. The pathophysiology of diabetes can be triggered by imbalances or disruptions in epigenetic mechanisms.

Small non-coding RNA sequences called microRNAs (miRNAs) are made when non-mature molecules are synthesized and processed in the nucleus and cytoplasm to become fully mature miRNAs. Upon maturation, miRNAs bind to the mRNA of their target gene, resulting in the silencing or degradation of the mRNA. The significance of miRNA-mediated post-transcriptional regulation in a variety of aspects of cell biology, including cell differentiation, cytokine and growth factor-mediated signaling, glucose metabolism, and insulin synthesis and secretion, is being highlighted by increasing evidence. T2DM can be caused by a direct impairment in the function of - cells caused by miRNA expression dysregulation. More than 2600 miRNAs have been identified in the human genome to date (miRBase, v.22.1), and several miRNAs, including miR-200, miR-7, miR-184, miR-212/miR132, and miR-130a/b/miR-152, have been shown to be involved in the pathogenesis of T2DM. By inhibiting genes like Snca, Cspa, and Cplx1 that are involved in vesicle fusion and SNARE activity, for example, miR-7 overexpression inhibits insulin secretion. Overexpression of miR-375 results in impaired exocytosis and decreased insulin secretion. On the other hand, the downregulation of miR-375 articulation causes a decrease in β-cell mass.

Post-translational histone methylation and the inclusion of non-canonical histone variants in octomers as part of the microRNA (miRNA) profile have been shown to persist even after normoglycemia restoration. MiRNAs partake in metabolic memory by focusing on the mRNA of qualities encoding chemicals engaged with DNA methylation and those firmly managed at the degree of advertiser methylation, record, and handling. High glucose levels have been shown to alter DNA methyltransferase activity and post-translational histone modifications (PTHMs), resulting in irreversible changes that explain the long-term negative effects of metabolic memory.

Hyperglycaemia actuates an overabundance of ROS age by mitochondria, which leads to diabetes entanglements that might endure in any event, when hyperglycemia is controlled. When good glycemic control is initiated very early, the damage caused by hyperglycemia-induced oxidative stress can be avoided, but if poor control is maintained for a longer period of time, it is difficult to reverse. Hyperglycemia, elevated oxidative stress, and excessive AGE formation are all linked in the early stages of T2DM. In addition to mitochondrial DNA damage, persistent protein glycation of respiratory chain components can result in a hyperglycemia-independent concatenation of events that synergizes oxidative stress and AGEs as the disease progresses. The impacts of this metabolic irregularity initiate provocative cycles through receptor restricting of AGEs or ROS which can change the arrangement and construction of the extracellular framework. Endothelial dysfunction and subsequent atherosclerosis may result from these structural changes.

At last, poor quality aggravation, which is associated with T2DM improvement and its vascular inconveniences, has been displayed to intercede metabolic memory. An inflammatory response that results in IR and endothelial dysfunction is triggered by a number of environmental factors that promote T2DM development, including age, obesity, sedentary behavior, and diet. Monocyte binding to endothelial and vascular smooth muscle cells, which in turn promotes monocyte-to-macrophage differentiation, is enhanced by obesity-related NF-B activation, which mediates the expression of inflammatory genes. Moreover, NF-κB enactment prompts articulation of provocative cytokines that are associated with vascular irritation, with ensuing age of endothelial grip atoms, proteases, and different middle people. The Toll-like receptor, which is linked to hypertension, insulin resistance, and obesity, is another important link between inflammation and oxidative stress in obesity.

In rundown, T2DM is a heterogeneous and moderate problem that addresses a progression of metabolic circumstances related with hyperglycemia and brought about by surrenders in insulin emission as well as insulin activity because of a complicated organization of neurotic circumstances. An increased risk of other diseases, such as heart, peripheral arterial, and cerebrovascular disease, obesity, and nonalcoholic fatty liver disease, among others, can be caused by a variety of different paths driven by a variety of genetic and environmental factors that interact and mutually reinforce one another.

Mitochondrial Dysfunction There is more and more evidence linking mitochondrial dysfunction to the onset of T2DM, age-related insulin resistance, and T2DM complications. Defective mitochondrial biogenesis, oxidative stress, genetic mutations that affect mitochondrial integrity, and aging all contribute to mitochondrial dysfunction and are closely linked to the development of type 2 diabetes.

ATP synthesis by oxidative phosphorylation in response to metabolic demand is the primary function of mitochondria. Additionally, mitochondria are involved in the production of various metabolites that serve as macromolecular precursors (such as DNA, lipids, and proteins). In addition, mitochondria integrate multiple signaling pathways and play an important role in ion homeostasis, ROS clearance, and the stress response. Mitochondrial dysfunction is a state that is characterized by a reduced ratio of energy production to respiration. Mitochondrial dysfunction is caused by an imbalance between energy intake and expenditure in the mitochondria. Under these conditions, supplement oxidation effectiveness is diminished prompting a diminished proportion of ATP combination/oxygen utilization, which expands O2− creation.

In point of fact, one suggested connection between mitochondrial dysfunction and IR is the accumulation of ROS in the mitochondria. Studies that found obese and insulin-resistant people had impaired lipid metabolism and mitochondrial oxidative capacity in skeletal muscle were consistent with this connection. Furthermore, patients with T2DM have been found to have downregulation of qualities associated with oxidative digestion that are managed by the peroxisome proliferator-initiated receptor γ co-activator 1α (PGC 1α) and a lessened phosphocreatine re-union rate, both characteristic of impeded mitochondrial capability. In addition, it has been discovered that some relatives of T2DM patients have decreased mitochondrial respiration, indicating that mitochondrial dysfunction may have existed prior to the onset of T2DM. As an alternative to a decrease in mitochondrial content, it has also been proposed that T2DM development may be the direct result of deficiencies in the electron transport chain (ETC) and the oxidative phosphorylation system.

The production of reactive oxygen species (ROS) is strongly linked to insulin resistance and mitochondrial dysfunction. ROS production increases when the ETC is unable to handle an excessive amount of electron input, primarily at complex I and complex III. As a result of nutrient depletion, electron supply to the mitochondrial electron transport chain (ETC) rises, and the excess electrons are transferred to oxygen, resulting in the production of oxygen and hydrogen peroxide. The Cys and Met residues in proteins are oxidized by ROS produced in mitochondria, resulting in damage to the protein's structure, impairment of its function, and ultimately cell death. ROS species also harm DNA and lipids in the membrane, which makes mitochondrial dysfunction worse. The polyol pathway is also triggered, which results in the production of AGEs, the expression of the AGEs receptor, and the ligands that activate them. Additionally, it contributes to the worsening of T2DM by activating PKC isoforms and upregulating the hexosamine pathway. In aggregate, unreasonable ROS age by mitochondria adds to sped up T2DM movement.

Mitochondrial brokenness remembers a decrease for mitochondrial biogenesis, alongside a lessening in the outflow of mitochondrial oxidative proteins, for example, and so on buildings, which prompts diminished substrate oxidation. Mitophagy processes are activated by damage caused by high oxidative stress in the mitochondria. Mitophagy is used to get rid of damaged mitochondria or, in cases of excessive cellular stress, to apoptosis. These two cycles diminish substrate usage and improve the collection of lipid intermediates, for example, diacylglycerols (DAG) and ceramide (CER) that upset the insulin flagging pathway. While CER inhibits protein kinase AKT, DAG increases IRS-1's serine/threonine phosphorylation, reducing its insulin-stimulated tyrosine phosphorylation and further propagating the insulin signaling pathway. In IR, mitochondrial dysfunction is caused by the accumulation of DAG and CER.

Downregulation of PGC 1, which has also been found in T2DM patients, may play a role in mitochondrial biogenesis defects. PGC 1α is a record coactivator that manages the statement of key qualities engaged with mitochondrial biogenesis, versatile thermogenesis and metabolic substrate digestion. In addition, PGC 1 is in charge of some of the oxidative metabolism-related genes that are downregulated in T2DM patients. In humans with T2DM, a key driver of mitochondrial biogenesis, mitofusin-2, is also downregulated. Interestingly, weight loss raises levels of mitofusin-2, indicating that mitochondrial dynamics defects are caused by an excess of nutrients and energy.

Through mitochondrial biogenesis and the selective clearance of damaged organelles, mitochondrial homeostasis is maintained. Mitochondrial elements are urgent to keeping up with sound mitochondria and control their amount. In a process known as mitophagy, which must be effectively and tightly regulated in order to preserve cell homeostasis, mitochondria fission encourages the removal of damaged mitochondria. As a result, mitophagy is thought to be one of the main mechanisms that control the quantity and quality of mitochondria. There are two steps involved in removing damaged mitochondria: the priming of damaged mitochondria for selective autophagy recognition and the induction of general autophagy. The products are then released back into the cytosol, where they are recycled as macromolecular components after the degradation process is finished. This process generates energy to protect the cell from stress and maintain cell viability in adverse conditions. Reduced hepatic insulin sensitivity and altered glucose homeostasis are two of the major pathological branches of Type 2 Diabetes (T2DM) development when mitophagy is impaired. As demonstrated by the onset of obesity and insulin resistance (IR) in mice following the ablation of fusion protein, deregulation of mitochondrial dynamics with a shift toward fission encourages metabolic dysfunction. In addition, in the C2C12 murine cell line and cybrids, respectively, increased mitochondrial fission and mitochondrial fragmentation have been linked to mitochondrial depolarization, impaired ATP production, decreased insulin-dependent glucose uptake, as well as increased mitochondrial ROS and impaired insulin signaling. These researches emphasize the detrimental impact that unbalanced mitochondrial dynamics have on metabolic health.

Fatty acid oxidation, a key metabolic defect in obesity and IR, is negatively impacted by enhanced mitochondrial fission, which also contributes to the accumulation of lipotoxic lipid species. Combination moved mitochondria elements has been likewise connected with an expansion in unsaturated fat usage putatively forestalling lipotoxicity.

The job of mitochondrial hereditary qualities in the gamble of T2DM has been plainly settled. Indeed, the development of T2DM has been linked to a number of mtDNA variants, both homoplasmic and heteroplasmic. A3243G, T14577C, and A5178C are the heteroplasmic variants currently linked to an increased risk of T2DM. The gathering of homoplasmic variations related with T2DM risk incorporates C1310T, G1438A, A12026G, T16189C and A14693G. It is essential to keep in mind that additional research is required to ascertain whether T2DM has an increased rate of mtDNA heteroplasmy in metabolically active tissues that produce more mitochondrial ROS.

To summarize, mitochondrial dysfunction and type 2 diabetes have a complex and bidirectional relationship. On one hand, parts of T2DM, for example, insulin obstruction can prompt mitochondrial brokenness, for example, through supplement overburden prompting ROS gathering. However, as evidenced by the presence of mtDNA variants associated with T2DM, mitochondrial dysfunction may predispose patients to subsequent T2DM. To better understand the connection between diabetes and mitochondrial health, more research is needed.

5. A decrease in the metabolic response of insulin-responsive cells to insulin or, at the systemic level, an impaired or lower response to circulating insulin by blood glucose levels is referred to as insulin resistance (IR). There are three main types of insulin-deficient or IR conditions: 1) decreased -cell insulin secretion; 2) insulin antagonists found in the blood, either as a result of non-hormonal bodies or hormones that counter-regulate; and, thirdly, an impaired response to insulin in the target tissues. In the fed state, the interaction of additional molecules like growth hormone and IGF-1 influences insulin's action. Glucagon, glucocorticoids, and catecholamines reduce the insulin response during fasting to prevent insulin-induced hypoglycemia.

Because it determines the relative degree of phosphorylation of downstream enzymes in the regulatory signaling pathways, the ratio of insulin to glucagon plays a significant role in this regulation. Glucocorticoids, on the other hand, encourage muscle catabolism, gluconeogenesis, and lipolysis, while catecholamines encourage glycogenolysis and lipolysis. As a result, IR may be caused by an excessive release of these hormones. Regarding the final category, there are three primary insulin-sensitive extra-pancreatic organs that are crucial to the aforementioned processes: liver, adipose tissue, and skeletal muscle. A deficient activity of insulin in these tissues frequently goes before the improvement of foundational IR, subsequently logically driving T2DM.

Skeletal Muscle

Skeletal muscle IR is viewed as the main extra-pancreatic consider the improvement of T2DM. By increasing plasma glucose uptake, insulin stimulates muscle glycogen synthesis under physiological conditions. Glycogen synthesis and glucose uptake are impacted by three primary rate-limiting factors:

glycogen synthase, hexokinase and the glucose carrier GLUT4. Upon insulin restricting to insulin receptor (INSR) in muscle cells, GLUT4 moves from intracellular compartments (early endosomes (EE), endosomal reusing compartment (ERC) and trans-Golgi organization (TGN)) to the plasma layer. This process reduces circulating glucose levels while facilitating glucose uptake.

A hyperglycemic state would result from mutations that reduce insulin receptor or GLUT4 expression as well as any defect in either the upstream or downstream signaling pathway. In order for insulin to influence glucose metabolism, it is necessary for INSR tyrosine kinase activity to be activated. When insulin binds to the INSR's -subunit, it phosphorylates the -subunit on a number of tyrosine residues, making it possible for insulin-mediated signaling. As a result, insulin action on skeletal muscle can be hindered by mutations in any of the main phosphorylation sites of INSR. In addition, mutations in phosphoinositide 3-kinase (PI3K) or other key proteins of the downstream signaling pathway, such as IRS-1 and IRS-2, impair insulin action on muscle. Environmental factors can also play a significant role in muscle glucose uptake, in addition to mutations or defective epigenetic regulation. Physical activity improves glucose utilization by increasing blood flow to skeletal muscle cells. IR and T2DM are both caused by obesity, which is associated with chronic inflammation. Increased immune cell infiltration and proinflammatory molecule secretion in intermyocellular and perimuscular adipose tissue may contribute to skeletal muscle inflammation, as evidence mounts. Through paracrine effects, this eventually results in myocyte inflammation, impaired myocyte metabolism, and IR.

Fat Tissue

Fat tissue is a metabolically unique tissue equipped for blending a great many naturally dynamic mixtures that control metabolic homeostasis at a foundational level. Indeed, adipose tissue is involved in a wide range of biological processes, including vascular tone control, appetite regulation, body weight homeostasis, coagulation, angiogenesis, fibrinolysis, reproduction, glucose and lipid metabolism, and immunity

Insulin follows up on fat tissue in two unique ways: (1) increasing triglyceride synthesis and glucose uptake; and (2) inhibiting triglyceride hydrolysis and encouraging the absorption of glycerol and FFA from the bloodstream. Glycolysis, which results in the production of glycerol-3-phospate (glycerol-3-P) and its incorporation into lipogenic pathways, is activated when GLUT4 is in the fed state, allowing glucose to be taken in by adipocytes from the bloodstream. The esterification of glycerol-3-P and the fatty acids from VLDLs results in the formation of triacylglycerol (TGA), which is stored in lipid droplets. In order to supply FFA that can be utilized as a source of energy in other tissues, TGA droplets in the adipocyte are depleted during metabolic stress.

Adipose IR (Adipose-IR) refers to adipose tissue's impaired response to insulin stimulation. Even in the presence of elevated insulin levels, adipose-IR can result in enhanced FFA release into plasma and impaired suppression of lipolysis. We discovered that adipose-IR affects a number of signaling components, including the activation of AKT, which prevents GLUT4 from translocating to the membrane and encourages the activation of lipolytic enzymes that cause hyperglycemia. As previously stated, adipose-IR is associated with glucose intolerance and elevated plasma FFA release, which accumulates in muscle and liver. FFA accumulation in the liver causes impaired insulin signaling, which leads to the development of type 2 diabetes (T2DM) and promotes hepatic gluconeogenesis and the impaired glucose-stimulated insulin response.

Pathologic vascularization, hypoxia, fibrosis, and macrophage-mediated inflammation are all correlated with abnormally increased adipose tissue mass. Saturated FFA-stimulated adenine nucleotide translocase 2 (ANT2), an inner mitochondrial protein that causes adipocyte hypoxia and activates the transcription factor hypoxia-inducible factor-1 (HIF-1), can be activated by obesity and a diet high in fat. Adipose tissue dysfunction and inflammation follow as a result. Hypertrophied adipocytes as well as fat tissue-occupant invulnerable cells add to expanded circling levels of proinflammatory cytokines. A chronic state of low-grade systemic inflammation, also known as metabolic inflammation, is facilitated by this increase in circulating proinflammatory molecules and local cytokine releases like TNF, IL-1, and IL-6. It is believed that this state of chronic inflammation plays a significant role in the pathogenesis of IR and T2DM.

Liver

In the liver, insulin doesn't just direct glucose creation/usage yet in addition influences lipid digestion all the more comprehensively. When pancreatic cells secrete insulin and circulating glucose levels rise, insulin binding to the liver INSR causes the receptor to become autophosphorylated. Insulin receptor substrates (IRSs) are subsequently recruited and phosphorylated as a result. Phosphatidylinositol (3, 4, 5)-triphosphate) is produced when phosphatidylinositol (4, 5)-bisphosphate (PIP2) is phosphorylated by IRSs, which in turn activate PI3K. The activation of PDK1 by PIP3 then phosphorylates AKT. Additionally, mTORC2 phosphorylates AKT. When AKT is completely actuated, it partakes in a few downstream pathways that direct various metabolic cycles including glycogen union, gluconeogenesis, glycolysis and lipid blend.

The precise control of hepatic glucose output is made possible in physiological states by the combined action of glucagon and insulin. Insulin is a potent inhibitor of glucose production when its concentration in the blood is elevated, whereas glucagon induces hepatic glucose production. There are both direct and indirect mechanisms at work when insulin affects the production of glucose in the liver. However, it is still unclear how important each of these mechanisms is in relation to the others.

Insulin inhibits hepatic glucose production by activating FOXO1, which reduces hepatic glucose release in addition to inducing glycogen synthesis. FOXO1 is a record factor that has a place with a subclass of the forkhead group of record factors that have a forkhead box-type DNA restricting space. On the promoters of the genes for glucose-6-phosphatase (G6Pase) and phosphoenolpyruvate carboxykinase (PEPCK), which both play important roles in maintaining glucose levels in states of starvation, FOXO1 recognizes a particular regulatory element known as the insulin response element (IRE).

In states of insulin resistance (IR), just like in tissues that are sensitive to insulin, hepatic cells do not respond to insulin in a manner that is appropriate. Glycogen synthesis in the liver is impaired, glucose production is not suppressed, lipogenesis is increased, and the synthesis of proteins like the pro-inflammatory CRP is increased. In fact, the liver's altered insulin response can be caused by an inflammatory state caused by the abnormal production of proinflammatory proteins like adipocytokines and cytokines and conditions like oxidative stress.\

Results and complications of T2DM: Cardiovascular Gamble

As depicted in the past segments, T2DM is a multisystem sickness with a solid relationship with CVD improvement T2DM is associated with both micro- and macro-vascular complications, the latter of which includes accelerated atherosclerosis leading to severe peripheral vascular disease, premature coronary artery disease (CAD), and an increased risk of cerebrovascular diseases T2DM also increases the adult mortality rate from heart disease and stroke by two to four times. T2DM is regarded as a significant risk factor for cardiovascular disease (CVD) due to these factors, most likely through the involvement of multiple molecular mechanisms and pathological pathways. These include how IR affects vascular function, atherosclerosis, oxidative stress, hypertension, the accumulation of macrophages, and inflammation.

Diabetic dyslipidaemia and the development of atherosclerosis Dyslipidaemia is a common symptom of type 2 diabetes, and it raises the risk of atherosclerosis and mortality in diabetics. A characteristic dyslipidaemic profile that includes elevated TG, TG-rich lipoproteins (TRLs), small dense LDLs (sdLDL), and decreased HDL levels is a sign of diabetes mellitus. Several factors, including hyperglycemia, insulin resistance, hyperinsulinemia, and abnormalities in adipokines and adipocytokines, have been implicated in the pathophysiology of dyslipidemia in T2DM. Experimental studies indicated a connection between cholesterol deposition and inflammation as a result of TRLs entering the artery wall and epidemiological studies indicated that TG-rich lipoproteins and their remnants contribute to atherogenesis and CVD risk. Numerous nascent and metabolically modified lipoprotein particles, such as liver-derived apoB100 (VLDL and its remnants) and intestine-derived apoB48 (chylomicrons and chylomicron remnants), make up TRLs. Size, density, and apolipoprotein composition of TRLs vary greatly.

Chylomicrons carry dietary lipids and lipid-biliary sources to the liver, where they acquire apoE, apo-CI, apo-CII, and apo-CIII from HDL upon entering central circulation. The hydrolysis of TG within the core of the chylomicron by Apo-CII, an activator of lipoprotein lipase (LPL), results in the release of free fatty acids (FFAs). Chylomicron remnants (CR) are formed as a result of the gradual removal of TGs and are cleared out by hepatocytes upon incorporation of. This, along with the take-up of FFA created by lipolysis in fat tissue gives the significant wellspring of hepatic VLDL gathering and discharge. Once in the dissemination,

VLDL particles consolidate apo-CII and apoE from HDL permitting VLDL to be continuously lipolyzed prompting the age of more modest VLDL particles (VLDL1, VLDL2 and VLDL3), IDL, lastly LDL. The metabolism, production, and elimination of lipoproteins are efficient processes. Mechanisms Leading to T2DM Dyslipidemia and Atherosclerosis Increased hepatic TG content in T2DM patients leads to elevated hepatic production of VLDL and normal or slightly elevated LDL-C levels, most commonly sdLDLs enriched in TG. However, T2DM and IR are among the most important metabolic derangements in these processes. They cause impaired metabolism and clearance of chylomicrons and VLDLs. Due to insulin's inability to inhibit hormone-sensitive lipase (HSL), impaired adipose tissue fat storage is one of the primary IR abnormalities. Adipocytes' intracellular TG stores release FFA continuously as a result. Hepatocytes take up the released FFAs, which can be directed to the mitochondria and oxidized there; be reabsorbed into TG in order to construct new VLDL particles; shifted to gluconeogenesis, which made hyperglycemia worse; or then again put away as TG prompting hepatic steatosis.

Increased liver production of VLDL-apoB100, particularly VLDL1, which is linked to insulin sensitivity indices, is the most common feature of diabetic dyslipidemia. This emphasizes the influence that insulin has on hepatocyte assembly and VLDL secretion. Almost every stage of VLDL assembly and secretion involves insulin. The microsomal transfer protein (MTP) gene, which codes for the protein that assembles TG with apoB100, is known to be inhibited by insulin. As apoB100 enters the ER lumen, MTP facilitates concerted lipid transfer, and lipidation determines the amount of the active pool of apoB100. Because lipidation of apoB100 is a co-translational process and a rate-limiting step in the stability of apoB100 mRNA, apoB100 degradation is caused by a lack of TG. The expansion of TG to apoB100 creates beginning VLDL particles that are shipped to the GA by Sar2/COPII-containing vesicles. VLDL maturation is facilitated by the phospholipase D1 (PLD1) within the GA. Accordingly, in insulin-safe condition, MTP articulation and movement is expanded subsequently adding to raising apoB100 lipidation and to its salvage from corruption. Indeed, acute insulin-mediated inhibition of apoB100 secretion is eliminated by IR.

The liver uses both de novo synthesized FAs and extra-hepatic FFAs as a substrate for TG synthesis, and the availability of TGs within hepatocytes is crucial for VLDL synthesis. In the fed state, where the sterol regulatory element-binding protein (SREBP) controls the expression of lipogenic genes, de novo lipogenesis takes place primarily. The SREBP-1c isoform up-directs practically every one of the proteins engaged with FA amalgamation as well as chemicals that supply acetyl-CoA units and diminishing counterparts to the pathway. The lipogenic effect of chronic hyperinsulinemia can be explained by the fact that insulin controls SREBP-1c. Adipose tissue-derived FFAs are another significant source of liver TGs and VLDL production. Adipose tissue production of FFAs rises in T2DM, as previously mentioned. Thusly, in IR, an expansion in TG lipolysis in fat tissue and FFA convergence fills in as one more wellspring of lipid to the liver.

As referenced above, in the IR milieu, insulin has decreased ability to hinder VLDL discharge in the fed express, the accessibility of apo-CII is lower and apo-CIII creation is expanded. Due to reduced TRL clearance by hepatocytes, these events cause the accumulation of VLDL remnants and IDL. LRP1 translocation from intracellular vesicles to the hepatocyte plasma membrane is also impaired by hepatic IR, which contributes to impaired TRL clearance.

In an effort to free TG from lipid residues (VLDL 2+3, IDL); RLPs), CETP is activated, promoting the exchange of TG between RLPs and HDL and LDL particles and incorporating CE from HDL and LDL. The TG-enriched HDL and LDL particles are better substrates for hepatic lipase lipolysis, which results in an increase in atherogenic sdLDL particles and decreased HDL-C levels in the blood. The expanded development of CE into circling TRLs intervened by upgraded movement of CETP assumes a key part in producing little thick HDL and LDL particles, the previous being less atheroprotective and the last more atherogenic. HDL clearance in the bloodstream is improved by TG enrichment.

The particle capacity of inducing cholesterol efflux from the cells, which is the first step in reverse cholesterol transport (RCT), is significantly reduced by the lower HDL concentration and altered HDL composition. In T2DM patients, flow-mediated vasodilation has been linked to impaired RCT activity and an increased risk of coronary artery disease (CAD).

The increased permeability of sdLDL into the subendothelial space accelerates atherosclerosis. Due to conformational rearrangements in apoB100 as the particle decreases in volume and size, SdLDL particles have a lower affinity for LDLR. Additionally, because sdLDL particles are more susceptible to oxidation, activated macrophages in the subendothelial space actively scavenge them for foam cells. Moreover, sdLDL particles show expanded proteoglycan restricting and worked with section into the blood vessel wall, expanded blood vessel maintenance, and a more drawn out half-life. Additionally, sdLDL particles are more susceptible to oxidation by free radicals, more resistant to breakdown, and more likely to be glycated.

The gene for apoA-I, the primary HDL particle apolipoprotein, contains an insulin response elemen. HDL biogenesis and apoA-I production decrease as insulin resistance in the liver increases. The ATP-binding membrane cassette transport protein A1 (ABCA1) is present in adipocytes. Adipocyte HDL formation is slowed by IR and ABCA1 expression is decreased on the surface. IR inhibits LPL, which reduces the amount of apoA-I released into the serum from chylomicrons. This highly atherogenic lipid profile is a key contributor to atherogenic dyslipidemia, which is causally linked to the development and progression of atherosclerotic cardiovascular disease (ASCVD). In addition, HDL particle concentrations tend to be dysfunctional and unable to perform their primary functions within the environment of insulin resistance (IR) in diabetes. Clinical evidence, genetic linkage studies, and prospective longitudinal cohorts all lend credence to the connection between atherogenic dyslipidemia and ASCVD. The INTERHEART study found that the apolipoprotein (apo) B100/apoA-I ratio, which represents the correlation between all apoB (atherogenic lipoproteins) and HDL (representing classically anti-atherogenic particles), was the best predictor of risk of myocardial infarction at the population level. Prospective randomized clinical trials utilizing statins have also demonstrated the connection between atherogenic dyslipidemia and ASCVD. Patients with atherogenic dyslipidemia have a higher risk of cardiovascular events than those without AD, even when treated with statins

In addition to other metabolic and vascular abnormalities, diabetes dyslipidemia increases vascular risk. Endothelial dysfunction is caused by a variety of mechanisms, including decreased vasodilation, increased vasoconstriction, increased free radical exposure, and impaired endothelial cell function, all of which contribute to the facilitation of pro-atherogenic conditions. It has also been found that oxidative stress goes up even more when the renin-angiotensin axis is active.

Endothelium plays a significant role in the regulation of vascular tone and structure through the balanced release of endothelial-derived relaxing and contracting factors. Impaired endothelial function and the onset of atherosclerosis. This equilibrium is adjusted in T2DM prompting modification of the physicochemical properties of the vascular wall by means of endothelial brokenness, oxidative pressure, platelet hyper reactivity, and aggravation. Atherosclerosis, thrombus formation, and increased vasoconstriction are all consequences of these abnormalities.

The passive diffusion of glucose through the plasma membrane of vascular endothelial cells makes them particularly vulnerable to the development of intracellular hyperglycemia in T2DM. Aldose reductase can activate the aldose reductase secondary metabolic pathway by metabolizing excess glucose in the sorbitol pathway to sorbitol and fructose in T2DM. At the same time, oxidation of NADPH to $NADP^+$ and reduction of NAD^+ to NADH occur simultaneously. Depleted NADPH and an elevated $NADH/NAD^+$ cytosolic ratio alter the redox potential, accelerating glycolysis and boosting DAG de novo synthesis. Nitric oxide (NO) levels drop and protein kinase C (PKC) is triggered as a result. Vascular permeability and contractility are increased as a result of these effects. Endothelial dysfunction is brought on by an increased NADH/NAD+ ratio, which also increases O2 production, LDL oxidation, cytotoxic effects on endothelial cells, and decreased NO availability.

The sorbitol pathway's excessive aldose production encourages protein glycosylation, which results in the stable Amadori products (like glycosylated hemoglobin) and AGEs. Several molecules are linked to AGEs, which increase oxidant activity and, as a result, ROS production. This causes more oxidative stress and prevents NO from being released, leading to vascular lesions. Endothelium-derived NO bioavailability and activity may also be diminished by AGEs, compromising vascular activity further. In addition, AGEs have the potential to induce receptor-mediated gene transcription, which in turn can cause endothelial activation and an inflammatory and pro-coagulant state. Endothelin-1, VCAM-1, ICAM-1, E-selectin, thrombomodulin, TF, vascular endothelial growth factor (VEGF), IL-1, IL-6, and TNF- are all transcribed following the activation of AGE binding to the RAGE-receptor. Expanded articulation of provocative and grip particles intensifies the fiery reaction and irritates diabetic vascular intricacies.

These favorable to fiery cytokines invigorate the articulation and arrival of supportive of coagulant particles and repress the declaration of hostile to coagulant atoms by endothelial cells. Increased growth factor production and a pro-coagulant state in the endothelium's surface cause the basement membrane to thicken, which favors protein and lipid deposition and inhibits vasodilation.

Hyperglycemia-associated vascular injury, oxidative stress, inflammation, and altered hemodynamic balance may initiate the development of atherosclerosis and the formation of arterial thrombus in T2DM. At the beginning of atherosclerosis, circulating LDL binds to matrix proteoglycans, where it is more likely to be oxidized. This results in highly pro-inflammatory particles that cause endothelial cells to express a number of adhesion molecules. Leukocyte transmigration into the vascular wall, as well as the recruitment and activation of circulating monocytes that differentiate into macrophages, are aided by this. A non-regulated mechanism by which macrophages remove the excess of oxidized LDL results in the formation of foam cells and the onset of fatty streaks. Inflammatory cytokines like IL-1 and IL-6 are released by mononuclear cells, which encourage the recruitment of additional inflammatory cells. Consequently, smooth muscle cells expand and migrate into the intima, where they produce and secrete extracellular matrix, which aids in the formation of fibroatheroma. Plaque fissures or ulcerations expose highly thrombogenic substances as the process progresses, resulting in platelet adhesion and aggregation, which in turn encourages the formation of thrombus. Likewise, platelets can likewise deliver favorable to fiery cytokines and development factors elevating monocyte enlistment to atherosclerotic plaques, which animates fibroblasts and smooth muscle cell expansion hence speeding up the atherosclerotic interaction.

A critical component of type 2 diabetes (T2DM) is a chronic low-grade inflammatory state known as "metaflammation". This condition is associated with diabetes and the progression of atherosclerosis. It has been proposed that this chronic condition is an underlying cause of the progression of atherosclerosis in T2DM. It involves the same cellular and molecular players as acute inflammatory responses and has been suggested as such. Hyperglycaemia can increment flowing cytokines that can prompt persistent aggravation in T2DM. In both monocytes and macrophages, patients with T2DM have higher levels of IL-1b, IL-6, IL-8, MCP-1, and other major cytokines. ROS-mediated activation of p38 and other proinflammatory kinases, upregulation of NF-kB induction, oxidative stress, and activation of the AGE-RAGE pathway are the underlying mechanisms involved in this process. In addition, the impaired phagocytic activity of macrophages caused by exposure to high glucose levels partially explains the higher prevalence of chronic infection in T2DM patients. Indeed, T2DM is linked to higher levels of IL-1 and IL-18, increased levels of the nucleotide-binding oligomerization domain-like receptor 3 (NLRP3), and increased inflammasome activity. Neutrophil extracellular trap activation, or NETosis, is the typical macrophage cell death that causes chronic inflammation. These markers have been found to be elevated in hyperglycemic states and to high levels in T2DM patients.

Adipokine Balance and the Risk of Cardiovascular Disease Adipose tissue dysfunction, which is one of the mechanisms of T2DM complications, can cause an imbalance between pro-inflammatory and anti-inflammatory adipokines. A number of studies have shown that adipokines are linked to insulin resistance (IR), can cause endothelial dysfunction, pro-inflammatory and pro-atherogenic states, and more.

Well-known as an insulin-sensitizing hormone, adiponectin's expression and circulating levels are inversely correlated with adiposity. Insulin-sensitizing properties are found in adiponectin. Adiponectin acts through ADIPOR1 and ADIPOR2 receptors and the peroxisome proliferator-actuated receptor α (PPARα) pathway, prompting diminished hepatic gluconeogenesis, expanded liver and skeletal muscle unsaturated fat oxidation, expanded glucose take-up in skeletal muscle and white fat tissue, and diminished white fat tissue irritation. Adiponectin also has strong anti-inflammatory effects on macrophages and fibro genic cells and prevents cell death by neutralizing inflammatory and lipotoxic ceramides and DAGs. Adiponectin levels that are low in T2DM patients are linked to an increased risk of developing premature arteriosclerosis, making them an additional risk factor for cardiovascular disease. Endothelial dysfunction, coronary artery disease, high blood pressure, and thicker carotid intima-media thickness are all linked to adiponectin deficiency. Low convergences of adiponectin lead to an expanded articulation of intercellular bond particle 1 (ICAM-1), vascular cell grip atom 1 (VCAM-1) and E-selectin, advances separation of macrophages into froth cells and improves the multiplication and relocation of smooth muscle cells.

Omentin is a white adipose tissue-derived adipokine that plays a role in glucose homeostasis. Omentin is present in the blood and is linked to lower levels in T2DM patients. Omentin has been shown to activate the AKT signaling pathway, enhancing insulin-stimulated glucose uptake in human adipocytes in vitro. Both at the protein and mRNA levels, omentin levels and IR are found to be inversely correlated in humans. Extra examinations show that omentin has calming properties, decreases cytokine articulation, and is adversely connected with fundamental fiery markers, for example, TNF and IL-6.

Vaspin (visceral adipose tissue-derived serine protease inhibitor) is an adipokine that prevents atherosclerosis and plaque formation by inhibiting the proteases that cause IR. Serum vaspin levels in T2DM patients are higher than those in healthy controls, it has been demonstrated. A 1.7-fold increase in CVD risk is linked to higher vaspin levels. Also, high vaspin is linked to more severe coronary artery disease. Conclusions: Research on diabetes, insulin, and glucose homeostasis is still very important. In fact, research on this topic must continue to expand as a result of rapid globalization, the normalization of a sedentary lifestyle, and an increase in obesity, diabetes, and the co-morbidities that come with them. To prevent, control, treat, or reverse the pathophysiology of T2DM and its complications, it is essential to comprehend the mechanisms involved in each step of the disease's development and complications. Early detection of T2DM through screening and intensive patient-centered management improves quality of life for patients, but more research is needed to figure out what causes the correlations between different demographic subsets and the corresponding variable risks for T2DM, as well as what causes people with low socioeconomic status to be at higher risk.

Precision medicine should be used with the help of molecular genetic tools to identify specific variants that contribute to the development of T2DM and to search for biomarkers to assess progression and response to therapeutic interventions, as the pathophysiology and underlying mechanisms of T2DM are becoming increasingly understood. To determine whether the intestinal microbiota plays a direct causal role in the pathogenesis of T2DM and how well treatments work, more research is needed.

It is abundantly clear that we still have a long way to go before we fully comprehend each of the numerous stakeholders in glucose homeostasis.

Pathophysiology of Hypertensive Renal Harm

Suggestions for Treatment

Dissimilar to most of patients with straightforward hypertension in whom negligible renal harm creates without extreme pulse (BP) rises, patients with diabetic and nondiabetic persistent kidney sickness (CKD) display an expanded weakness to try and direct BP heights. An impairment of the renal autoregulatory mechanisms that normally reduce the transmission of elevated systemic pressures to the glomeruli in uncomplicated hypertension is the cause of this increased susceptibility, according to research conducted in experimental animal models. The particularly lower BP edge for renal harm and the more extreme slant of connection among BP and renal harm in such states requires that BP be brought into the normotensive territory down to forestall moderate renal harm. The renal protection provided by renin-angiotensin system (RAS) blockade is proportional to the BP reduction in animal models when BP is accurately measured using radiotelemetry, with little evidence of BP-independent protection. Critical analysis of the clinical data also suggests that RAS blockade's BP-independent renoprotection has been overemphasized, and that lowering BP targets is more important than choosing an antihypertensive regimen. However, due to their propensity for salt retention, CKD patients without aggressive diuresis struggle to achieve these BP goals. A more compelling justification for the use of RAS blockade in the treatment of CKD patients than any alleged BP-independent renoprotective superiority is the effectiveness of RAS blockers in lowering BP in patients who have been adequately treated with diuretics and their potassium- and magnesium-sparing effects.

The overall gamble of serious renal harm in patients with simple fundamental hypertension is low as contrasted and other cardiovascular complications.1,2 By and by, given the gigantic commonness of hypertension in everyone, it actually stays the subsequent driving reason for end-stage renal sickness (ESRD), with the gamble being considerably higher in blacks.2 By and large, hypertension-prompted renal harm in patients with straightforward fundamental hypertension has been isolated into the 2 unmistakable clinical and histological examples of "harmless" and "dangerous" nephrosclerosis.3 Harmless nephrosclerosis is the example seen in most of patients with straightforward essential hypertension. To some degree vague vascular injuries of hyaline arteriosclerosis grow gradually without unmistakable proteinuria. Albeit central ischemic glomerular obscelence and nephron misfortune happen after some time, renal capability isn't genuinely compromised besides in helpless people, for example, blacks in whom the cycle will in general follow a more extreme and sped up course. "Malignant" nephrosclerosis, on the other hand, is associated with very severe hypertension (the malignant phase of essential hypertension) and has a distinctive renal phenotype of acute disruptive vascular and glomerular injury accompanied by significant fibrinoid necrosis and thrombosis. Vascular damage frequently results in ischemic glomeruli. In the absence of appropriate treatment, renal failure can develop rapidly. Although episodes of malignant nephrosclerosis unquestionably contribute to the development of ESRD in patients who are not treated, who do not adhere to treatment, or who abuse cocaine, the full-blown clinical phenotype has thankfully become rare due to the widespread availability of effective antihypertensives.

Recognizing that the spectrum of hypertension-induced renal damage includes both benign and malignant nephrosclerosis is a significant development over the past two decades. There is a lot of evidence that coexisting hypertension is a major factor in the progression of most chronic kidney diseases (CKDs), including diabetic nephropathy, which is currently the leading cause of end-stage renal disease (ESRD).3–5 These negative effects are observed even with mild to moderate elevations of blood pressure (BP) in CKD patients, indicating an increased vulnerability to hypertensive renal damage, a lower BP threshold for damage, and a steeper slope of the Due to the lack of a specific histological phenotype, it has been difficult to quantify the contribution of hypertension to progressive renal disease. In this setting of CKD, vascular pathology, which is thought to be the hallmark of hypertensive injury, is frequently absent. Instead, the underlying renal disease's intrinsic phenotype appears to be superimposed on an accelerated segmental or global glomerulosclerosis (GS).

Pathophysiology of Hypertensive Renal Damage the degree to which any vascular bed is subjected to the elevated pressures is likely to determine the direct negative effects of hypertension. As a result, the three broad categories of pathogenetic determinants of hypertensive renal damage are as follows: 1) the foundational BP "load"; 2) the extent to which this load reaches the vascular bed of the kidney; what's more 3) neighborhood tissue defenselessness to some random level of barotrauma. It appears to be plainly obvious that on the grounds that the encompassing BP profile in cognizant creatures is portrayed by unconstrained, quick, and frequently enormous changes in BP, traditional secluded BP estimations are innately lacking to characterize quantitative connections among BP and renal damage.5-8 The accessibility of BP radiotelemetry by permitting persistent BP checking in cognizant excessive creatures has given a meaningful step forward in hypertensive objective organ harm research.

BP Burden and Its Transmission to the Renal Microvasculature

Regularly, expansions in foundational BP, long winded or supported, are kept from completely coming to the renal microvasculature by proportionate autoregulatory vasoconstriction of the preglomerular vasculature with the end goal that renal blood stream and glomerular hydrostatic tensions (PGC) are kept up with moderately steady. As a result, these autoregulatory responses serve as the primary safeguard against hypertensive renal damage.5, 10 Only benign nephrosclerosis is observed as long as blood pressure stays below a certain threshold (within the autoregulatory range); A clear illustration of such a threshold relationship between BP and malignant nephrosclerosis has recently been demonstrated using BP radiotelemetry in the stroke-prone spontaneously hypertensive rat model. Moreover, as would be predicted, even modest BP reductions to below this threshold were shown to prevent such damage.13 In general, chronic hypertension tends to shift both the upper and lower limits of autoregulation to the right and represents a protective adaptation.5,14 Therefore, an acute severe elevation in BP

However, increased transmission of elevated systemic pressures to the renal microvasculature can result in renal damage even in the absence of severe hypertension. It is anticipated that any significant preglomerular vasodilation will result in a greater fractional transmission of the ambient systemic pressures, after uninephrectomy or in early type 1 diabetes (before significant nephropathy).

On the other hand, only a modest increase in the risk of hypertensive injury is expected if this vasodilation is not accompanied by impaired renal autoregulation or severe hypertension.15 This may account for the generally benign renal course in most uninephrectomized individuals and possibly the long delay in the development of overt diabetic nephropathy.15,16 On the other hand, if renal autoregulation is also impaired, as seen after more severe (75 pattern C) shows a significantly increased risk of hypertensive injury due to the steeper relationship between blood pressure and kidney damage and the significantly lower BP threshold for damage. Additionally, in the absence of hypertension severe enough to cause vascular injury, this enhanced glomerular pressure transmission primarily results in accelerated GS...

Through the use of BP radiotelemetry, it has been demonstrated that the progressive GS of the initially normal remnant glomeruli in these rats follows the quantitative relationships with the significance of autoregulatory capacity as a determinant of the susceptibility to hypertensive injury is further illustrated by the effects of the dihydropyridine calcium channel blockers (CCBs) in this model. The rat 5/6 renal ablation model is the model these agents, not surprisingly, further impair renal autoregulation in the 5/6 ablation model, given the critical dependence of autoregulatory response on voltage-gated calcium channels. Similar adverse effects of dihydropyridine CCBs and protective effects of a low-protein diet on GS have also been noted in the streptozotocin-induced diabetes model. Of note, differences in autoregulatory efficiency have also been postulated to account for some of the strain (genetic) differences in susceptibility to hypertensive injury. However, it needs to be emphasized that these adverse effects of impaired renal autoregulation on susceptibility to hypertens. When systemic pressures are reduced in a vasoconstricted bed, impaired autoregulation primarily results in a decreased capacity to maintain renal blood flow and glomerular filtration rate (GFR), which increases the risk of ischemic tubulointerstitial injury. Local BP-Independent Determinants of Tissue Susceptibility Although still poorly defined, differences in the severity of damage expressed at any given degree of increased pressure exposure (barotrauma) may result from genetic or acquired differences in intrinsic structure or function. For instance, there is evidence that glomerular hypertrophy may be an independent risk factor for In addition to the expected increase in wall tension (Laplace Law: It has been hypothesized that the glomerular capillary epithelial cell (podocyte) provides structural support against pressures that are significantly higher than those in systemic capillaries (45 versus 20 mm Hg) through its interdigitating foot processes Hypertrophy of glomerular capillaries may also compromise their ability to withstand mechanical stress. tension=pressureradius). During glomerular hypertrophy, this terminally differentiated cell may have limited replication potential, limiting its capacity to maintain mechanical support and physical integrity under hypertensive stress.

However, the most attention has been paid to the BP-independent tissue damage-promoting effects of angiotensin II and, more recently, aldosterone.4,12,24,27–29 Oxidative stress and the activation of growth factors and fibro genic mediators like transforming growth factor- and plasminogen activator inhibitor-1 are hypothesized to result from the activation of several downstream deleterious cellular and molecular pathways. The majority of studies in animal models have claimed to show glomeruloprotection by renin-angiotensin system (RAS) blockade and/or aldosterone antagonists over and beyond that achieved by "equivalent" BP reductions with other antihypertensive regimens. However, when BP has been measured more continuously by radiotelemetry instead of intermittently by tail-cuff, the renoprotection can be entirely With RAS blockade, neither a shift to a higher BP threshold for damage nor a decrease in the slope of the relationship between BP and GS are observed. This is in contrast to what would be expected with significant protection that is independent of BP. In this unique circumstance, it is applicable to take note of that confined PGC estimations like segregated BP estimations may not precisely reflect constant tension openness. Even in models with excellent correlation with systemic BP measured by radiotelemetry, there is no consistent correlation between PGC and GS24 due to these limitations.

These results, taken as a whole, suggest that angiotensin II and/or aldosterone alone may not trigger the activation of downstream molecular mediators of tissue injury; rather, it may be a response to tissue stress and/or injury in and of itself. There is proof that pressure alone can enact a considerable lot of these downstream pathways, and the histological aggregate of hypertensive renal harm shows little contrast in models regardless of unmistakable RAS activation.

On the other hand, little proof of the enactment of these pernicious pathways or renal harm is seen without raised pressures in spite of significant angiotensin and aldosterone increments during low salt admission, congestive cardiovascular breakdown, or cirrhosis, or in the cut kidney of the 2-kidney-1-cut model of Goldblatt hypertension.36 as a matter of fact, the organization of even exceptionally a lot of exogenous aldosterone brings about little objective organ harm in creatures kept up with normotensive on a low-salt eating regimen. In addition, studies of aldosterone's pathogenicity have typically failed to account for changes in potassium balance, which can also have an effect on renal damage.37 As a result, although it is still possible that angiotensin II and aldosterone may amplify hypertensive renal damage through BP-independent mechanisms in particular situations and/or models, definitive evidence has yet to be obtained.

Unresolved Problems Despite the progress that has been made, there are still some fundamental problems with hypertensive target organ damage. Although recent clinical data have indicated that systolic and possibly pulse pressures are more closely correlated with target organ damage than mean arterial or diastolic pressures, 1 the pathophysiological basis of such empirical observations remains unknown, which is why the term "BP load" is used as a generic term. The relative pathogenic importance of individual BP parameters—

mean, systolic, diastolic, pulse pressure, and BP variability—remains undefined. Additionally, it is possible that the relative pathogenic potential of each of these BP parameters may differ depending on the target organ. In addition, individual BP fluctuations must be transmitted in accordance with their rate (frequency) and the kinetics of autoregulatory responses in order for fluctuating systemic pressures to be transmitted to target organs in real time. Additionally, pressure transients and/or peak pressure fluctuations in the microvascular system may be more pathogenic than long-term elevations. This protective function seems to be supported by the unusually rapid activation kinetics of the afferent arteriolar myogenic response that have recently been observed[38]. Additionally, the fact that systolic rather than mean blood pressure appears to be the trigger signal for this response[38] may indicate that systolic (peak) pressures have a greater potential to cause disease. The potential for renal microvascular transmission and the pathogenic significance of these individual components of BP power (energy/unit time) are being evaluated with the help of biophysical approaches that are being developed to separate the BP energy into its component parts.

Therapeutic Implications Based on the discussed pathophysiology of hypertensive renal damage, there are three main therapeutic targets: 1) lowering the BP load; 2) lessening the transmission of pressure to the renal microvasculature; furthermore (3) interference or potentially alteration of the nearby cell/sub-atomic pathways that intervene possible tissue injury and fibrosis.

Reduction of BP Load Given the substantial evidence that local hypertension (barotrauma) is a major contributor to the onset and progression of renal damage, it stands to reason that treating the proximate cause of these elevated pressures—i.e., effectively lowering the systemic arterial pressures—would be the most effective preventive strategy. However, the clinical context will determine the relative success of such BP reductions in preventing renal damage. In patients with straightforward hypertension, even modest and simple BP reductions below the autoregulatory threshold are likely to prevent malignant nephrosclerosis.[5, 13] On the other hand, in CKD patients, BP may need to be lowered well into the normotensive range to prevent additional GS. The more restricted accomplishment against moderate renal sickness as contrasted and dangerous nephrosclerosis and hypertensive stroke is subsequently not unexpected.1, 2 The systolic BP objective of 140 to 150 mm Hg that was thought of as OK up to this point in patients with CKD, on the grounds that regardless of whether accomplished, it probably won't have been sufficiently low to forestall proceeded glomerular barotrauma. The pathophysiology of hypertensive glomerular injury in these states predicts that the further developed the CKD (the more prominent the vasodilation and autoregulatory debilitation), the lower the accomplished BP should be to standardize intrarenal pressures.

Even within the CKD population, the impact of BP reductions may differ due to intrinsic differences in susceptibility due to disease cause and severity, as well as genetic and environmental factors.5,7,8 The steeper the slope of the relationship between BP and renal damage, the greater the impact of any given BP reduction. Furthermore, even transient episodes of

BP elevations are predicted to be more freely transmitted to the glomerular capillaries, suggesting the need for around-the-clock BP control.39 The recognition Because proteinuria may be a biologic marker of enhanced intrinsic glomerular susceptibility or may reflect increased glomerular pressure transmission, it is not surprising that proteinuric CKD patients experience greater benefits from aggressive BP control40.

The claims for the therapeutic superiority of RAS blockade have not been sustained, at least for cardiovascular disease and stroke, most recently by the very large landmark ALLHAT trial.1, therefore, recent guidelines now stress the primary importance of BP reductions per se in preventing target organ damage. Patients with CKD, however, remain a notable exception, with continued emphasis on RAS blockade as the initial regimen of choice. These recommendations are based on the results of several randomized controlled clinical trials in

However, a critical review of the clinical trial data reveals that the interpretations are not as clear-cut, and the BP-independent benefits of RAS blockade that have been emphasized are much smaller than previously thought. This problem is shown by the Collaborative Study Group's reexamination of the landmark clinical trial in type 1 diabetic nephropathy patients. A very impressive 50% RR reduction was reported by RAS blockade (25 renal end-points in 207 captopril-treated patients versus 43 in 202 conventionally treated controls). Nearly all of the end-points and RR reductions were observed in the higher-risk patients who had a serum creatinine of these large RR reduction estimates were said to not be significantly altered by statistical adjustment for these differences, despite the control group's greater proteinuria at entry and the captopril group's smaller but statistically significant differences in BP throughout the course. However, the validity of the parent study's interpretations is seriously questioned by a substudy of the 108 nephrotic patients considered to be at greatest risk that was later published49. This substudy showed that these high-risk nephrotic patients had been disproportionately randomized, with 42 patients entering the captopril group and 66 patients entering the placebo group (P 0.002 by 2). The fact that only eight of the 100 nonresponders, whose average serum creatinine more than doubled throughout the study, experienced remission from proteinuria and also showed significant BP reductions, confirming the high risk status of these patients (7 in the captopril group) Of note, of the 16 dark nephrotic patients, none of whom answered, 14 were appointed to the benchmark group (P<0.03). The erroneous randomization of the 24 nephrotic patients who were at very high risk to the placebo group probably largely explains the difference in 18 additional end-points between the control group and the original report.

The more recent IDNT and RENAAL trials of angiotensin receptor blockers (ARBs) in type 2 diabetic nephropathy provide some insight into the relative magnitude of the BP-dependent versus BP-independent effects of RAS blockade.46,47 The additional renoprotection (slower decline in GFR) provided by ARBs compared with control antihypertensive regimens was 1 mL/min per year (5 16 BP reductions in the conventionally treated groups, on the other hand, reduced the rate of GFR decline by 6 mL/min per year, despite the fact that untreated patients' GFR decline rates have historically been 12 mL/min per year. As a result, the antihypertensive effects of ARBs may account for up to 85% of the overall benefit. In addition, the fact that the achieved clinic BP in the RAS blockade-treated groups, as in other clinical trials in diabetic and nondiabetic nephropathy patients, tended to be 2 to 4 mm Hg lower than in the control groups raises questions about the BP independence of even this residual additional renoprotection by ARBs. It is possible that such differences in clinic BP reflect larger differences in ambient and/or nocturnal BP, as revealed in a HOPE substudy.50 Reductions of 3/2 mm Hg in clinic pressures in a subset of 38 ramipril-treated patients translated into a reduction of 10/4 mm Hg in an average 24-hour ambulatory BP (ABP) in the same patients because of a large decrease in nocturnal BP of 17/8 Subsequently, as in creatures, BP-free impacts of RAS bar are challenging to show while ABP checking is used,5,8 proposing a requirement for alert while surmising BP autonomy dependent exclusively upon center tensions, which are generally not controlled for the hour of day as well as relationship to medicate dosing. Even though intermittent 24-hour ABP monitoring may not provide as complete an assessment of the total chronic BP burden as is possible with radiotelemetry in experimental models, its incorporation in future clinical trials, at least in subsets of patients, should be strongly considered. This is because diabetic hypertensive patients frequently do not exhibit the normal nocturnal decline in BP. Given the data from the experimental animals, it is not surprising that significantly better correlations are observed between 24-hour ABP measurements and markers of cardiovascular target organ damage

When comparing antihypertensive regimens, caution must also be exercised when drawing conclusions regarding BP-independent effects. The superior renal outcomes with RAS blockade compared with CCBs in the AASK trial[48] may in fact reflect the adverse effects of CCBs on BP transmission to the microcirculation.[20,21] However, it should be acknowledged that unlike rodent models, the evidence for deleterious effects of dihydropyridine CCBs in humans for hard end-points, rather than proteinuria, is more mixed.[52] This may reflect the limitation of clinic BP measurements combined with the fact that Additionally, the detrimental effects of

CCBs may not be relevant to more proximal vascular injury and may only be significant in accelerated GS models where the capillary bed is the primary site of injury. There is reason to suspect that at least some of this difficulty has stemmed from an underuse of aggressive diuretic use in these patients,53 in part because of some justifiable concerns about their adverse impact on renal function parameters.54 However, hypertension in most CKD patients is volume-dependent with relative RAS suppression and exhibits an increased BP salt sensitivity because of altered pressure natriuresis.55,56 As a consequence, BP reduction by agents other than diuretics usually tends to Such pathophysiology makes sense of why monotherapy in CKD patients, incorporating that with RAS blockers, is for the most part insufficient. Therefore, effective diuresis is usually required to maintain adequate BP control in CKD patients, and some hemodynamically mediated elevations in blood urea nitrogen and creatinine levels are unavoidable and may need to be considered acceptable unless they are severe. The fact that diuretics and RAS blockers counteract each other's side effects on potassium and magnesium balance but are synergistic for BP reductions makes their combination a logical antihypertensive regimen for these patients. Effective diuresis also activates the RAS and restores the antihypertensive effects of RAS blockade.57 In point of fact, a stronger case can be made for using RAS blockade to achieve BP objectives than for any protection that purports to be independent of BP. Reduced potassium and magnesium depletion in diuretic-treated patients may partly account for some of the BP-independent beneficial effects of RAS blockade and Aldactone's relatively low doses on cardiovascular morbidity and mortality in congestive heart failure patients.

As previously mentioned, it is theoretically possible to reduce hypertensive renal damage through nonantihypertensive interventions like protein restriction by hemodynamically reducing the intrarenal transmission of systemic pressures. However, in contrast to its effectiveness in rodent models, the benefits in clinical trials have been relatively modest and only discernible in patients with more advanced renal disease.59 The reasons for this are still unknown, but it is possible that the effect of dietary protein will only become quantitatively significant after a significant loss of functional renal mass and autoregulatory capacity.

Other pharmacological agents that preferentially vasoconstrict the preglomerular vasculature have the theoretical potential to decrease PGC and GS as well. Nonsteroidal anti-inflammatory drugs and cyclosporine A, on the other hand, are limited in their clinical utility due to their propensity to exacerbate hypertension and their risk of tubulointerstitial disease. Preglomerular vasodilation can hopefully be reduced and autoregulatory capacity increased without adverse effects, according to current research. In a similar vein, it might soon be possible to independently alter the molecular mediators of tissue injury that follow. To completely halt the progression of CKD, such additional interventions may be required. Given the increased fractional BP transmission in these patients, even if complete systemic arterial normotension is clinically achieved, it may not be sufficient to completely normalize glomerular hydrostatic pressures.

Conclusions Recent research has shed light on the pathogenesis of hypertensive renal damage and revealed that the degree to which renal autoregulatory mechanisms fail to prevent BP elevations from reaching the renal microvasculature determines how severe the damage is. Patients with diabetic and nondiabetic chronic kidney disease (CKD) may be more susceptible to progressive renal damage with even moderate hypertension if these protective mechanisms are impaired. Additionally, this kind of damage to the kidneys is likely to kick off a vicious cycle of hypertension that will be harder to break, resulting in even more nephron loss and increased glomerular pressure transmission. As a result, recent guidelines acknowledge that the primary clinical strategy to break this cycle remains achieving normotension in CKD patients, despite its difficulty. When BP load was accurately assessed using radiotelemetry, there was little evidence in experimental animal models for the much-hyped BP-independent protection by RAS blockade. In a similar vein, the clinical evidence is also less conclusive than previously stated. In any case, the debate is more scientific than clinical practice-related. RAS blockers are very effective antihypertensives in effectively diuresed CKD patients, and the majority of CKD patients require aggressive diuresis to achieve BP control. In the majority of CKD patients, this antihypertensive synergy and their counteracting effects on potassium and magnesium balance support the use of combined diuretics and RAS blockades. In any case, focusing on BP-independent mechanisms to prevent hypertensive renal damage is likely to have a greater impact on the still-escalating incidence of ESRD than finding more effective methods to achieve the lower BP goals.

Pathophysiology of bradykinesia in Parkinson's sickness

Bradykinesia implies gradualness of development and is one of the cardinal appearances of Parkinson's infection. Bradykinesia may be caused by weakness, rigidity, or tremor, but none of these factors fully explain it. We contend that the failure of basal ganglia output to reinforce the cortical mechanisms that prepare and carry out movement commands is the cause of bradykinesia. Midline motor areas exhibit the cortical deficit to its greatest extent. This prompts specific trouble with independent developments, delayed response times and strange pre-development

EEG movement. Usually-timed EMG bursts are used to perform movements, but the amount of EMG activity isn't enough to achieve the desired movement parameters. Sensorimotor integration and sensory scaling are also affected. The cerebrum has all the earmarks of being ready to remunerate somewhat for the basal ganglia shortfall. During task performance, the lateral premotor areas are overactive, and sensory cues can speed up movements. It is also beneficial to pay attention to movement. On the other hand, we suggest that engaging compensatory processes may also result in lower performance on other tasks. Patients' difficulties with multitasking, for instance, may be caused by a lack of resources to both compensate for their basal ganglia deficit and perform two tasks simultaneously. It is unlikely that surgical treatments will only be effective if basal ganglia output is normalized to that of healthy individuals. It seems more likely that surgery removes an interfering signal, allowing other structures to compensate more effectively.

Introduction James Parkinson first coined the term bradykinesia to describe one of the hallmarks of the disease that is now known as Parkinson's. However, bradykinesia may be a component of motor dysfunction in many movement disorders, as is now understood.

Two additional terms are frequently used interchangeably with bradykinesia: akinesia and hypokinesia. While akinesia refers to a lack of spontaneous movement (such as facial expression) or associated movement (such as arm swinging while walking), strictly speaking, bradykinesia refers to the slowness of a performed movement. Frozenness and taking a long time to move are two additional manifestations of akinesia. Hypokinesia refers to movements that are not only slow but also smaller than expected, like the micrographia in patients' handwriting. Even though these three symptoms are related, they must also be separate to some extent because individual patients may not have a good correlation between them (Evarts et al., 1981). Patients with Parkinson's disease frequently appear clumsy, which is likely caused by multiple aspects of the motor disorder.

We'll refer to all of these issues with slowness or lack of movement as "bradykinesia" in this review.

However, we will always define the specific functional deficits that we believe are relevant to each case when we believe that distinct mechanisms are involved. It will be helpful to first take into consideration other secondary factors that can contribute to bradykinesia before discussing the central mechanisms of bradykinesia and how they relate to the dysfunction of the basal ganglia that lies at the heart of Parkinson's disease.

Secondary causes of bradykinesia In Parkinson's disease, there are five potential causes of bradykinesia. Muscle weakness, rigidity, tremor, variation in movement, and a slowing of thought are all symptoms.

Numerous researches (Stelmach and Worringham, 1988; Stelmach and other, 1989; Jordan and other, 1992) have compared the strength of healthy age-matched subjects and Parkinson's disease patients. Even though this did not always reach statistical significance, they all observed a slight decrease in strength across a variety of muscle groups. It is challenging to match patient and control groups in terms of daily exercise and diet, which may account for this lack of agreement.

Corcos and colleagues recently attempted to address this issue by measuring elbow strength in patients while ON and OFF L-dopa following overnight therapy withdrawal (Corcos et al., 1996). Maximum elbow extension strength decreased by 30% and elbow flexion strength decreased by 10% when the patient stopped taking the medication. The difference in strength must have been caused by patients' inability to fully engage their elbow muscles because intrinsic muscle properties could not have changed during the brief interval between the OFF and ON conditions. Lack of volitional drive was not considered a factor in that study because the patients appeared to be highly motivated to produce strong contractions when receiving ON and OFF therapy. Brown and colleagues found that the persistence of action tremor during maximal contraction was one physiological reason for the strength loss in wrist extensors in a subsequent study (Brown et al., 1997). Patients receiving OFF therapy may experience tremors with a frequency of less than 10 Hz because it prevents maximum fusion of motor unit contractions and may contribute to weakness. Nonetheless, this can't represent the reduction in strength in all muscle gatherings, so other, probably focal, factors should likewise be involved. The conclusion is that Parkinson's disease patients may be weak in certain muscle groups, which will invariably result in slow movement.

It is unclear whether attention could influence strength testing results. Patients' inability to fully energize their muscles, especially when they are not receiving drug treatment, only indicates that they lack some of the normal voluntary input to the lower motor centers. It is unclear why this occurs. There is no conspicuous absence of exertion by patients and there doesn't have all the earmarks of being any absence of focus. Patients frequently state that they are working as hard as they can. In a similar vein, the fact that patients and healthy people have physiologically distinct EMG activity suggests that the voluntary drive to contract is not organized in the same way as usual. Nonetheless, peculiarities, for example, perplexing kinesia propose that there are components that can conquer this clear absence of volitional drive yet this is most likely not a consideration related peculiarity.

Inflexibility

Long-idleness stretch reflexes are improved in Parkinson's sickness (Tatton and Lee, 1975; Berardelli and others, 1983; Rothwell and others, 1983). If they were elicited in an antagonist muscle during an active isotonic contraction of the agonist, they could possibly contribute to bradykinesia. Using a torque motor to stretch muscles unexpectedly during active sinusoidal wrist movements, Johnson and colleagues tested this hypothesis (Johnson et al., 1991). They demonstrated that the degree of abnormality was related to the amount of clinical bradykinesia and that reflexes elicited in the antagonist muscle were not suppressed as much as they were in normal subjects. The fact that the antagonist muscle did not engage in any more activity than normal subjects did during unperturbed flexion/extension movements was the only flaw in this argument. Therefore, antagonist co-contraction did not appear to be a limiting factor in the actual movements tested. Even in very rapid movements, where the triphasic ballistic movement EMG pattern has been studied in detail, co-contraction has never been mentioned as a key feature. The conclusion must be that no conclusive evidence exists for the role that rigidity plays in bradykinesia.

Rest and action tremor

As mentioned earlier, Parkinson's disease weakness can be exacerbated by action tremor. Rest and action tremor both have the potential to lengthen reaction times. According to Hallett and colleagues and Wierzbicka and colleagues, Parkinson's disease patients typically time the onset of agonist muscle activity at the elbow or wrist with the time that the same muscle is activated in any ongoing tremor (Hallett et al., 1977; Wierzbicka et al., 1993). On average, this could stymie the beginning of any movement.

Voluntary alternating movements can be sped up or slowed down by action tremor. When patients attempt to move at frequencies close to those of their natural action tremor, Logigian and colleagues demonstrated that voluntary movements are entrained by action tremor (Logigian et al., 1991). The amplitude of the patients' ongoing tremor determines the extent of the entrainment.

Variability in movement Parkinson's disease patients' movements are less accurate than normal, especially when they have to move quickly (Sanes, 1985; 1990, Sheridan and Flowers; Phillips and others, 1994). To put it another way, the trade-off between speed and accuracy is less effective in patients than it is in healthy people. According to Sheridan and Flowers (1990), bradykinesia may be the result of patients' active strategy to move more slowly in order to improve accuracy. Bradykinesia persists in tasks where spatial accuracy constraints have been removed, making this a plausible strategy (Teasdale et al., however). 1990).

Bradyphrenia, or thought slowness, can interfere with movement planning and, for example, increase reaction time, which can cause bradykinesia. There has been debate regarding the existence of bradyphrenia in Parkinson's disease. This is in part because many Parkinson's patients do develop dementia from multiple causes, and dementia is characterized by a slowing of thought (Berry et al., 1999). Alteration in thought and depression are also associated with aging (Cooper et al.,, 1994), and these variables should be thought of. Finally, a lot of "cognitive" studies have used procedures that require a motor response, making it possible for bradykinesia to cause apparent bradyphrenia (Rafal et al., 1984). Numerous studies that did not take these factors into account have caused confusion. In addition, thinking isn't just one process; the speed at which it occurs may also be affected by the nature of the task. Cooper et al., some studies have claimed to find bradyphrenia. 1994; the majority, however, have not (Rafal et al., 1994). 1984; Duncombe and group, 1994; Howard and other, 1994; Spicer and others, 1994). When dementia is not present and the patient is not taking medications that could affect cognitive processes, such as anticholinergics, it is likely that bradyphrenia is not to blame for the slowing.

All of the aforementioned factors can cause bradykinesia, but they must be distinguished from the fundamental disorders of central movement control that cause primary bradykinesia. The characteristics of bradykinesia that cannot be explained by secondary factors are discussed in this section.

Bradykinesia could be brought on by a lack of speed in either formulating or carrying out the instructions to move (programming). Although programming and execution are typically viewed as distinct and sequential processes, they may overlap, at least to the extent that programming may continue while execution is being carried out. It is conceivable, consequently, to concentrate on a portion of the cycles engaged with programming in the event that we keep ourselves to estimations, for example, response times or EEG/attractive encephalography (MEG) concentrates on made before the beginning of developments. After the start of the movement, measurements may show execution as well as programming.

Getting ready to move: studies of reaction times Akinesia is caused when people with Parkinson's disease react more slowly than healthy people their same age. Response times decrease with disease progression. It is unclear whether patients are having difficulty preparing the instructions to move or releasing those instructions, which would explain their slow start to movement.

Comparing reaction tasks in which the amount of preparation is variable but the movement component is constant yields some information about preparatory processes. Healthy individuals are able to fully prepare the response in advance of the imperative signal in a straightforward reaction task. The response is influenced by the reaction signal in a choice reaction task. Subjects are aware of the possible actions they may need to take, but they are not aware of the specific actions required for any given trial. They must complete additional preparation after the crucial signal is given because they are unable to fully prepare the movement in advance. Choice reaction times are consequently longer than simple reaction times.

Parkinson's disease causes slower simple reaction times (Heilman et al., 1976; Evarts and other, 1981; Rafal and co., 1984; Bloxham et al., 1987; Sheridan and others, 1987; 1990, Hallett; Jahanshahi et al., 1992, 1993; Kutukcu and other, 1999; see additionally Zimmerman et al., 1992; Harrison and other, 1993; Revonsuo and other, 1993). With choice reaction times, the situation is more complicated. According to Varts et al., some authors have stated that they are the same as normal. 1981; Bloxham et al., 1987; Sheridan and others, 1987) and have proposed that patients' slow simple reaction times are caused by their failure to fully program their responses in advance. However, other authors (Wiesendanger et al.,) have reported that choice reaction times are longer than normal. 1969; Stelmach and other, 1986; Mayeux and others, 1987; Dubois and other, 1988; Lichter and others, 1988; Reid et al., 1989; Pullman and others, 1988; Jahanshahi and others, 1992; Brown and others, 1993b). The reason for the wide range of results reported is unclear. Some might emerge on the grounds that different patient gatherings were learned at various phases of the illness; some may be caused by aspects of the task's design, like stimulus–response compatibility, which may be handled differently in Parkinson's patients (e.g., Brown et al., 1993b). There is evidence that patients are likely to be slower than normal in preparing expected responses, regardless of whether they can fully utilize prior programming (Jahanshahi et al., 1992).

There is much clearer evidence, in contrast to the disagreement regarding the extent of programming deficits in Parkinson's disease, that slowness in executing motor commands is a significant factor in extending reaction times. The reason for this is that before movement or even EMG activity can be detected, motor excitability must reach a certain threshold. The threshold is reached later than usual if this is slow. Patients' EMG activity, for instance, typically increases slowly after its onset, which can delay movement detection. The same argument can be made for the time before EMG starts: Before motor neurones are discharged, motor excitability must reach a threshold. Pre-movement excitability increases more slowly than normal in Parkinson's disease patients, as demonstrated by experiments using magnetic transcranial stimulation (Pascual-Leone et al., 1994). The conclusion is that difficulties initiating the commands to move account for only a small portion of the increase in simple reaction times. The deficiency emerges either on the grounds that some unacceptable (slow) orders have been picked or on the grounds that the right orders are executed more leisurely than typical.

These studies on reaction time have led us to the conclusion that problems with the execution of a stored motor command are just as much to blame for slow performance in simple reaction tasks as it is for keeping that command in storage in the right state of readiness. More research is needed on the choice of reaction tasks situation.

Getting ready to move: EEG, MEG, PET, functional MRI (fMRI), and magnetic stimulation techniques have all been used to try to figure out which parts of the motor system in akinetic Parkinson's disease patients are acting abnormally. Studies of motor activity, on the other hand, have focused on the time immediately preceding movement, when changes in sensory input are minimal, because brain activity during movement reflects both outgoing motor commands and the sensory input that results from moving. In many examples, the developments are independent; response undertakings include pre-development tactile information that can muddle the translation of the information got. These studies generally indicate that midline (supplementary motor cortex (SMA) and nearby areas) cortical motor areas are underactive, possibly in conjunction with increased activation of lateral premotor areas. The first possibility is that it has to do with having trouble writing moving instructions; the latter may be an active process of compensation and may be connected to the performance boost that results from using external cues to direct movement (more on this below).

Before the start of a self-paced voluntary movement, the pre-movement EEG potential, also known as the Bereitschaftspotential (BP), is a slowly rising negative potential that appears over a large portion of the scalp. There are two main parts to it. The early component, also known as BP1 in this context but with other names, begins between one and two seconds before movement. It is symmetrical on both sides and is largest at its vertex. The second component, also referred to as NS1 or NS' in this instance but with a steeper rise, begins approximately 650 milliseconds prior to the onset of EMG activity. According to recent recordings obtained from subdural electrodes, the BP1 primarily reflects bilateral activity in the motor and supplementary motor areas, whereas the BP2 also incorporates activity from the contralateral motor and premotor cortex (Ikeda et al., 1992).

In the early studies, there was some debate about whether Parkinson's disease patients had elevated blood pressure. Dick and colleagues showed that L-dopa could affect the amplitude of the BP in both patients and healthy people, and that the difference between Parkinson's disease patients and healthy people was largely determined by the level of dopaminergic function (Dick et al., 1989). They continued by demonstrating that the BP of patients OFF therapy was lower in the beginning (BP1) but higher than normal later (BP2) (Dick et al., 1989). In the end, the patients' peak BP was almost identical to that of normal people. They suggested that the early component was reduced due to underactivity of a source in the SMA, which was compensated for by over activity in lateral motor areas closer to movement onset. Recent research tends to back up this idea. For instance, Jahanshahi and colleagues found that Parkinson's disease patients' pre-movement EEG activity was normal when they performed an externally triggered task, in contrast to the decrease in self-paced movements (Jahanshahi et al., 1995). According to Cunnington and colleagues, Parkinson's disease patients who under activated the SMA were more reliant on external cues and did not use predictive models when cues were available. 1995,

1997). However, if patients were asked to pay attention to the time of the next movement, pre-movement activity could be induced, which improved task performance (Cunnington et al., 1999). According to the authors, attentional processes make it possible for lateral premotor systems, which are less affected by dysfunction in the basal ganglia, to make up for deficits in midline motor systems, which are usually active in tasks that are generated internally.

The subjects did the same movement over many trials in these early studies. In later studies, the participants were required to select between a variety of actions—such as moving a joystick up, down, left, or right—on each trial. The fact that healthy subjects have a much higher BP than those who perform the same movement each time may be due to the additional processing required to choose between movements on each trial (Touge et al., 1995; Praamstra and others, 1996a, b, 1998; Dirnberger and others, 2000). Praamstra and associates utilized dipole demonstrating to show that the most probable hotspot for the additional actuation was the SMA (Praamstra et al., 1996b). This additional enactment is deficient in patients with Parkinson's sickness, predictable with the model framed previously.

Irregularities in cortical enactment before and during development have been likewise found with the method of occasion related desynchronization (Defebre et al., 1996; Magnani et al., 1998). EEG activity in the alpha (10 Hz) and beta (20 Hz) ranges decreases less than one second before movement begins and remains lower than at rest throughout movement. Cortical neurones' activity tends to become synchronized during periods of relative inactivity, which may explain the 10–20 Hz rhythm. If this is the case, event-related desynchronization is a sign of cortical activation that shows the population's activity breaking up into more distinct patterns in time and space. The pattern of movement-related attenuation of the alpha and beta rhythms during various motor tasks is abnormal in Parkinson's disease patients, and the duration of the event-related desynchronization prior to voluntary movements is shorter. According to Brown and Marsden's findings from 1999, dopaminergic stimulation can restore movement-related attenuation of the alpha and beta rhythms in Parkinson's patients. This effect was correlated with an improvement in bradykinesia and was specific to the motor areas involved in the motor task. In their study of simple and complex movements, Wang and colleagues found similar results (Wang et al., 1999). According to the preceding research, voluntary movement necessitates the release of cortical components from idling rhythms by the basal ganglia. Brown took this idea one step further in a recent study by examining the effect of dopaminergic stimulation on the coupling of activity between various basal ganglia nuclei (Brown et al., 2001). When they recorded the local potentials of patients who had electrodes implanted in the subthalamic nucleus and internal pallidum, they discovered that when the patients were not taking their medication, they were coupled by activity at 20–30 Hz, while when they were taking their medication, this changed to 60–70 Hz.

Motor execution In Parkinson's disease patients, single ballistic movements at a single joint are slower than normal. Single movements made as quickly as possible about a single joint (for a review, see Berardelli et al., and 1996a). While the agonist muscle's weakness may account for some of this slowing, other factors must account for the majority. For instance, although the speed of elbow flexion may decrease by half in the OFF condition, the maximum biceps contraction strength decreases by 10%. In a similar vein, the EMG data indicate that the antagonist does not exhibit excessive co-contraction, which could have slowed the movement more than was anticipated due to the decrease in strength. Instead, it appears that difficulties in rapidly recruiting the appropriate level of muscle force are to blame for slow movement.

There are two sections to this issue. To begin with, patients might find it hard to quickly enact a muscle. In cases of disease that have advanced: Some patients may require several seconds to produce a maximum voluntary contraction (Corcos et al., 1996). However, bradykinesia in simple movements isn't just caused by the rate of contraction. The fastest movements are accompanied by a triphasic EMG pattern in which the amplitude and other movement parameters determine how quickly and long the bursts last. Patients with Parkinson's disease exhibit this pattern, but the initial agonist burst is brief. According to Hallett and Khoshbin (Hallett and

Khoshbin, 1980), as a result, patients frequently add additional bursts of EMG to the pattern in order to achieve sufficient force to move the limb to the required end position. Despite this, the agonist burst's size may increase if patients aim for a movement of greater amplitude. This essentially indicates that the size of the agonist burst does not always limit movement slowed down: The speed would have been normal if the burst for the larger movement had been used for the smaller one. The conclusion is that simple movement bradykinesia has a second cause: improperly scaling the dynamic muscle force to the parameters of the movement (Berardelli et al., 1986b).

Movements that are simultaneous, sequential, or repetitive if a simple movement is made more complicated by repeating it or combining it with other tasks, bradykinesia becomes more apparent. This phenomenon is frequently utilized in clinical tests for bradykinesia. According to Agostino et al., repetitive sequential movements involving isolated finger movements, hand opening/closing, or wrist pronation/supination become smaller (hypokinesia) and slower (fatigue) with repetition. 1998). Patients were instructed by Schwab and colleagues to squeeze a sphygmomanometer bulb with one hand and draw an outline with the other (Schwab et al., 1954). If they had to complete both tasks at the same time, they had much more trouble than if they had to do them separately. In fact, patients tended to alternate between the tasks rather than perform them simultaneously in the majority of cases.

These characteristics of bradykinesia have been thoroughly examined in experimental studies. They demonstrate, in essence, that bradykinesia is more than just the slowness of single movements. Combining or maintaining complex movements presents additional challenges. Benecke and colleagues looked at rapid elbow flexion movements in conjunction with hand movements performed simultaneously or sequentially with the same arm or the opposite arm (Benecke et al., 1986, 1987). Patients with Parkinson's disease showed (i) a marked slowing of movement above and beyond that seen in each task alone when both had to be performed together, and (ii) a longer pause between each element of a sequential task, as opposed to normal subjects, in whom there was no decrease in performance when two tasks were combined. In fact, these two additional deficits had a better correlation with clinical bradykinesia measures than each simple movement's slowness.

Bilateral reaching has been associated with similar difficulties in performing simultaneous movements (Stelmach and Worringham, 1988; Castiello and Bennett, 1997), and tasks involving cranking 1998). In everyday movements, such as getting up from a chair to pick something up or drinking from a cup, there have been long pauses between each element in sequential movements (Bennett et al., 1995). Longer-lasting movement sequences have also been associated with fatigue (Berardelli et al., 1986a; Agostino and others, 1992, 1994).

What are these additional deficits in complex movement performance?

The issue of switching between tasks or combining them is not limited to movement. It can be seen in cognitive or motor-cognitive tasks at the same time (Brown and Marsden, 1991; Oliveira and other, 1998). These kinds of observations are important because they show that the extra deficit seen in complex movements isn't always just a motor issue. They raise the possibility that attention-involved global processing mechanisms are also a factor. According to Brown and Marsden (Brown and Marsden, 1991), patients either have a limited processing resource that prevents them from simultaneously working on multiple tasks or have difficulty switching this resource between tasks. An alternative is that patients use the same global resource but perform tasks less automatically than normal subjects. In this scenario, each task would use up more processing power, making it difficult to complete multiple tasks at once or switch between them. Actually, patients might be attempting to make up for absence of basal ganglia input by dedicating more assets to each single undertaking they perform. This becomes a constraint when needed to complete multiple tasks at once.

Sensorimotor processing A few authors have mentioned that Parkinson's disease can cause problems with sensorimotor processing. Two-point discrimination accuracy and proprioceptive position sense precision decreased, according to Schneider and colleagues (Schneider et al., 1986), and

Klockgether and colleagues suggested that Parkinson's disease patients have impaired peripheral afferent feedback in a study of arm movements that tested the effects of both visual and kinaesthetic information (Klockgether et al., 1995). Demirci and colleagues (Demirci et al.,) demonstrated a difficulty in matching somatosensory and visual inputs. 1997). The authors hypothesized that this was caused by an abnormal scaling of sensory information and made comparisons to the abnormal scaling of motor output that Berardelli and colleagues reported (Berardelli et al., 1986b).

Precision grip/lift tasks may also reveal a deficit in sensorimotor integration. These are mind boggling acts that are performed by holding an item with the right measure of power so it doesn't fall between the fingers when it is taken off a supporting surface. Peak grip force development takes longer in Parkinson's patients, and the rate at which grip force is generated significantly slows down. Additionally, when they lift the object into the air, they squeeze it more than usual (Fellows et al., 1998). The authors believed that issues with sensorimotor processing were to blame for the latter effect. Kinaesthesia may play a role in

Parkinson's disease pathophysiology, but its significance remains unclear, we conclude.

Sensorimotor processing abnormalities can also be used to explain contingent negative variation (CNV) anomalies. Between a warning (S1) and an imperative (S2) stimulus, the CNV is a slow negative potential. It reflects processes related to planning a forthcoming movement and anticipating the crucial stimulus and is best recorded at frontal and central electrodes. Movement of the prefrontal cortex adds to the abundancy of the CNV. In Parkinson's sickness, the abundancy of the CNV is decreased by a sum connected with the seriousness of illness and levodopa therapy (Amabile et al., 1986; Ikeda et al., 1997; Gerschlager and others, 1999). As a rule, the CNV is more plainly impacted in Parkinson's illness than the (single development) BP. This may be due to the following factors: S2 serves as a trigger for the final movement in a CNV task, whereas there is no trigger in a self-paced task. Therefore, patients OFF therapy can still rely on S2 as an external trigger to retrieve the instructions to move even if they fail to prepare for the upcoming movement in the S1–S2 interval. Because there would effectively be no contribution from processes involved in movement preparation, such conditions would significantly reduce the CNV. In contrast, preparation must have been completed prior to the movement in a self-paced task; As a result, the impact on the CNV will always be greater than that on the BP.

The corticomotoneurone connection is normal in Parkinson's disease, according to transcranial stimulation studies using electrical and magnetic stimulation techniques (Dick et al., 1984). In fact, whether the stimulus is given to patients who are immobile and receiving OFF therapy or dyskinetic and receiving ON therapy, the movements that are elicited by direct stimulation of the motor cortex are the same. This indicates, as previously stated, that a deficit in the motor cortex's final output pathways is not the primary cause of bradykinesia. Despite this, cortical stimulation has revealed minute alterations in the circuits of the cortex. Some of these may be compensatory while others may cause bradykinesia.

According to the majority of authors, Parkinson's disease patients' motor cortex has the same threshold for stimulation as healthy subjects (Priori et al., 1994;

Valls-Solè and others, 1994; Ridding and others, 1995). However, the normal slope of the input–output relationship between stimulus intensity and response size is steeper when patients are tested while at rest. According to Valls-Solè et al., voluntary contraction may facilitate responses less than in normal subjects. 1994). the implication is that the cortical excitability distribution at rest is skewed toward higher than normal values. This could be the result of a deficit in the primary basal ganglia, but it also seems likely that it is an effort to make it easier to recruit activity from a resting state in order to make up for the slow recruitment of commands to move.

The excitability of cortical inhibitory circuits also changes. During the subject's tonic voluntary contraction, a suprathreshold stimulus causes a muscle twitch, which is followed by a postexcitatory silence. According to Fuhr et al., the activation of cortical GABAergic inhibitory systems that suppress motor cortical output for 100–200 milliseconds is thought to be the cause of the disappearance of voluntary activity during the silence period. 1991). Bradykinetic patients have a shorter silent period (Cantello et al., 1991; Priori and others, 1994), and L-dopa treatment brings it back to normal (Priori et al., 1994). The double-pulse paradigm developed by Kujirai and colleagues (Kujirai et al.,) can also be used to test cortical inhibition in still subjects. 1993). Again, patients exhibit less inhibition than usual (Ridding et al., 1995). A different kind of abnormality is found when the interstimulus intervals are long and the conditioning and test stimuli are larger (suprathreshold). At 100 and 150 milliseconds, the test response is significantly slowed down (Berardelli et al., 1996b); this suggests that Parkinson's disease patients are less able to facilitate voluntary muscle activation. Reduced facilitatory input from basal ganglia to the cortical excitatory and inhibitory circuits could explain these effects on inhibition and excitation. In bradykinesia, the rate at which cortical motor output is recruited could be affected by either.

Recent transcranial magnetic stimulation studies have demonstrated that it is sometimes simpler to disrupt motor cortex activity in patients than in healthy subjects. Cunnington and colleagues, for instance, demonstrated that while single-pulse stimulation over the SMA may have no discernible effect on healthy subjects, it may disrupt task performance in patients early before movement begins (Cunnington et al., 1996). Patients' compromised activity is probably more easily disrupted than usual in the midline cortical areas.

Metabolic imaging (PET and fMRI studies) Consistent with the electrical data above, metabolic studies reveal a relative underactivation of midline motor areas in many tasks, occasionally accompanied by an increase in lateral premotor area activation. The studies provide more information about the specific cortical areas involved than EEG or MEG, but a unique paradigm must be used to differentiate between preparation and execution.

Many examinations have utilized a self-guided joystick development task in which subjects pick on every preliminary which bearing to climb, (down, left or right). The anterior SMA, anterior cingulate cortex, dorsolateral prefrontal cortex, basal ganglia, and thalamus are less activated in patients than in healthy subjects when compared to rest (Jenkins et al., 1992; Playford and other, 1992; Rascol et al., 1992; Jahanshahi et al., 1995). The selection or programming of a new movement on each trial is linked to activity in the anterior SMA and the dorsolateral prefrontal cortex, according to experiments on normal subjects (Deiber et al., 1991, 1996). As a result, the idea that producing or selecting the appropriate commands for a forthcoming movement is a fundamental component of bradykinesia is supported by the fact that patients' underactivation of these areas. Indeed, measures of bradykinesia are improved while underactivation in these areas is reduced when apomorphine is injected (Jenkins et al., 1992; Rascol and others, 1992). Dyskinetic patients exhibit frank over activity of the SMA as well as the ipsilateral and contralateral primary motor areas (Rascol et al., 1998).

Intriguingly, there is evidence that bradykinetic patients' sequential finger movements activate other parts of the cortex more than usual. Extra activation in the lateral premotor and parietal cortices was described by Samuel and colleagues (Samuel et al., 1997a). Sabatini and associates, utilizing fMRI as opposed to PET, revealed comparative outcomes however with extra actuation additionally in the caudal SMA, the foremost cingulate and, surprisingly, the essential sensorimotor cortex (Sabatini et al., 2000). Similar findings were obtained when Catalan and colleagues examined the performance of lengthy sequences of finger movements (Catalan et al., 1999). They discovered that as movement sequences became longer or more complex, activity in the ipsilateral cerebellum, as well as in the primary sensorimotor, premotor, and supplementary motor cortex, increased in healthy individuals. The premotor and parietal cortices were more active in patients than in healthy individuals. The conclusion is that the primary basal ganglia deficit may be compensated for by additional movement-induced circuit recruitment by the parkinsonian brain.

Bradykinesia and other diseases of the basal ganglia
In Parkinson's disease, slowness of movement (bradykinesia) is accompanied by a decrease in spontaneous movement (akainesia or hypokinesia). However, hyperkinesia and bradykinesia coexist in Huntington's disease and dystonia, two other basal ganglia disorders. This suggests that bradykinesia operates in a different manner than hypo- or

hyperkinesia. However, an examination of the bradykinesia's nature reveals that even this one symptom may have multiple causes. In patients with either dystonia or Huntington's disease, the maximum speed of simple voluntary arm movement is slower than in healthy subjects (Hefter et al., 1987; Thompson and others, 1988; van der Kamp and others, 1989; Berardelli and others, 1998, 1999), but the pattern of EMG activity that underlies the sluggishness in movement in patients with either of these conditions differs from Parkinson's disease patients. EMG bursts are frequently prolonged in dystonia and Huntington's disease, and the final position and peak velocity are more variable than in Parkinson's disease.

Additionally, Huntington's disease sufferers are unable to perform simultaneous and sequential movements normally (Thompson et al., 1988; Agostino and others, 1992) and have difficulty performing a sequence of movements without external cues, just like Parkinson's disease patients (Georgiou et al., 1995).

Test Parkinsonism and Examples from Medical Procedure

Most of the basal ganglia yield, especially that in the 'engine circle' (Albin et al., 1989; Alexander and Crutcher 1990a; Alexander and others, 1990b), via the thalamus, projects back to the cortex. GABAergic and inhibitory, the internal globus pallidus and the substantia nigra pars reticulata are the projection neurones of the main output nuclei. In the late 1980s, when the current model of basal ganglia function was being developed, it was hypothesized that the amount of observable movement was directly correlated with the discharge level in the output nuclei, with a high discharge causing hypokinesia and a low discharge causing hyperkinesia (Wichmann and De Long, 1996). This idea seemed to be supported by a number of observations. Microelectrode recordings made during neurosurgery suggested that the same might be true in human Parkinson's disease patients (Hutchinson et al., 1990). When monkeys were made parkinsonian by injecting MPTP (1-methyl-4-phenyl-1, 2, 3, 6-tetrahydropyridine) (DeLong, 1990), the level of resting pallidal discharge increased (DeLong, 1990). 1997). Indeed, pallidal neurones' firing rate decreased when apomorphine was injected to treat bradykinesia during Parkinson's disease surgery (Hutchinson et al., 1997; Merello and other, 1999). The latest accounts from patients going through pallidotomy for hemiballism or dystonia additionally propose that, in these hyperkinetic conditions, pallidal neurones fire at rates significantly not exactly those saw in patients with Parkinson's sickness (Lenz et al., 1998; Vitek and co., 1999).

Nonetheless, a basic connection between the degree of pallidal action and development can't completely make sense of probably the main consequences of stereotaxic medical procedure. This was referred to as "the paradox of stereotaxic surgery" by Marsden and Obeso (Marsden and Obeso, 1994). Pallidotomy has been used to treat several hundred patients worldwide since its revival in the early 1990s. However, lesioning this major basal ganglia output does not result in hyperkinesias, as might have been expected if there were strict correlations between movement and pallidal output. In actuality, the opposite is the case: After several years of L-dopa treatment, the drug-induced dyskinesias that are common can be reduced or even eliminated with pallidotomy. Even hyperkinetic basal ganglia disorders like dystonia and hemiballism have been successfully treated with pallidotomy (Lozano et al., 1997; Suarez and other, 1997; Vitek and co., 1999). Pallidotomy only has a slight effect on bradykinesia or hypokinesia, despite its success in treating or preventing hyperkinesia. There is only a 30% improvement in clinical bradykinesia scores in Parkinson's disease patients who are not receiving L-dopa treatment, and there is virtually no effect on clinical scores evaluated in the best ON condition (e.g., Samuel et al., 1998).

There are two main types of explanations that attempt to explain this fundamental paradox: ii) changes in neural noise-related physiological abnormalities; and (ii) anatomical explanations because the output structures of the basal ganglia are so intricate. It is currently impossible to determine which of these explanations is correct.

According to the physiological (neural noise) explanation, the mean level of discharge from the substantia nigra pars reticulata and globus pallidus internus is not the only important physiological measure of basal ganglia function. It is likely that the output's absolute level, as well as its temporal and spatial pattern, is relevant. According to Mink (1996), this pattern may assist in focusing cortical activation so that appropriate muscles are activated and others are suppressed while performing a task. It is theorized that this result becomes confused in Parkinson's sickness. There is unquestionably a rise in the temporal variability of pallidal discharge in parkinsonian monkeys and human patients treated with MPTP, as well as a tendency for the discharge to be more synchronized between distant cells than in the healthy state (Bergman et al., 1998).

It is reasonable to speculate that pallidotomy cuts off the thalamus's connection to a chaotic and noisy system. The 30% improvement in clinical scores after receiving OFF treatment could be explained by the fact that bradykinesia was caused by a single pattern of noise. Lesioning would also eliminate dyskinesias that were caused by another pattern. However, the fact that there is no suggestion that lesioning the pallidum normalizes basal ganglia function is the most significant aspect of this development of the basal ganglia model—and one that is frequently overlooked by those who use it. The newer model views lesioning as a means to completely eliminate basal ganglia output, in contrast to the simple model, which views lesioning as a means to normalize the overall level of pallidal output. The implication is that if the lesion improves function, it must be because other parts of the brain are better able to compensate for the usual contribution from the basal ganglia. This proposition is investigated underneath.

The physical answer for the mystery of pallidal medical procedure is that the game plan of pallidal yield is more complicated than had been conceived initially (for a survey, see for example Parent and Hazrati, 1995). Particularly suggestive are the effects of chronic high-frequency stimulation of the globus pallidus internus, which resembles a reversible lesion. The electrodes that are typically inserted have four different stimulation points that make it possible to activate various parts of the globus pallidus internus. Krack and colleagues discovered, employing this method, that the globus pallidus internus is divided into two distinct functional zones (Krack et al., 1998). Although stimulation in the ventral zone improved rigidity and reduced drug-induced dyskinesias, it also eliminated L-dopa treatment's anti-akinetic effects. OFF-drug bradykinesia was improved by stimulation near the border of the globus pallidus internus and the globus pallidus externus, but dyskinesias were also possible in some patients. On the off chance that consequences for bradykinesia and dyskinesias can be isolated physically, it is conceivable that the underlying model of basal ganglia capability can in any case be applied. Bradykinesia can be reduced by reducing output in one part of the system, while dyskinesias can be eliminated by interrupting function in another part of the loop. This theory still holds that normalizing basal ganglia output rather than completely removing it is the cause of improvement in motor function, in contrast to the previous physiological explanation.

At this point, it would be helpful to learn more about how surgery affects Parkinson's disease patients' bradykinesia. The findings suggest that surgery may result in both improved compensation and normalized function.

Deep brain stimulation and neurophysiological studies of surgery's effect on bradykinesia a lot of clinical studies have looked at how well pallidotomy works; chronic stimulation of the subthalamic nucleus or globus pallidus has received relatively little attention. However, in terms of bradykinesia, pallidotomy typically results in an improvement of 30% in OFF-period symptoms on the side opposite the lesion that persists for at least two years following the procedure. The best ON-therapy scores and measures of postural stability are less affected (Bronstein et al.,, 1999; Lang and others, 1999). Pallidal feeling makes comparative impacts, yet is viewed as possibly more secure with regards to unfriendly mental incidental effects in the event that respective methods are performed (Brown et al., 1999). When it comes to reducing OFF-treatment bradykinesia scores, chronic stimulation of the subthalamic nucleus may be more effective than pallidotomy or pallidal stimulation. Additionally, improvements in posture and balance are more apparent (Limousin et al., 1998). In most cases, dyskinesia issues can be alleviated by lowering the dose of L-dopa.

In an effort to gain a deeper comprehension of the nature of the improvement that these procedures produce in patients who are not receiving their usual drug therapy, a number of studies have combined clinical measurements with physiological techniques. The majority of the time, the main improvement is in execution rather than movement preparation. Therefore, pallidotomy and stimulation of the subthalamic nucleus both increase the recruitment of maximum muscle force and speed up both simple and complex movements (Pfann et al., 1998; Brown and others, 1999; Kimber and other, 1999; Limousin and other, 1999; Siebner and other, 1999). However, reaction times are significantly reduced, and the BP1 (early) component of the blood pressure) is unaffected (after pallidotomy; Limousin and other, 1999). It is interesting that the late (BP2) portion of the BP is improved, which is consistent with the idea that surgery may improve compensation by non-midline cortical structures.

The model of basal ganglia function that was presented in the early 1990s has been the driving force behind many functional imaging studies of the effect that surgery and deep brain stimulation have on bradykinesia. Overactivity of the inhibitory result projections from the basal ganglia to the thalamus in Parkinson's sickness should eliminate facilitatory thalamocortical drive, especially to midline cortical engine regions (foremost SMA and cingulate cortex). Pallidotomy was anticipated to improve activation by restoring normal levels of basal ganglia output (e.g., Ceballos-Baumann et al., fMRI activation studies had shown that these areas were less activated during movement in patients...

Similar findings have been reported in the majority of studies on movement-related changes in metabolic activity both before and after pallidotomy (Grafton et al., 1995; Samuel, 1997a, b), as well as during stimulation of the subthalamus (Limousin et al., 1997; et al., Ceballos-Baumann 1999). Increased activation of the dorsolateral prefrontal cortex is typically accompanied by increased activation of the preSMA and anterior cingulate cortex in free-choice joystick movement tasks. Albeit most reports of enactment prompted digestion propose that there is no adjustment of the essential engine cortex, there are a few ideas that excitement of the subthalamic core might diminish action in the resting state (Limousin et al., 1997; et al., Ceballos-Baumann 1999). It is unknown whether this is connected to a general decrease in rigidity or other involuntary muscle activity or to decreased input to the cortex via pathways that originate directly from the subthalamus.

Even though premotor areas are not typically underactive in Parkinson's disease and may even be overactive, surgery appears to also increase their activation. Both a comprehension test (Grafton et al.,) and a 1995) and in a joystick movement task that was chosen at random (Ceballos-Baumann et al., 1999). Eidelberg and colleagues found increases in metabolism in the premotor cortex, dorsolateral prefrontal cortex, and motor cortex ipsilateral to a pallidotomy in a fluorodeoxyglucose-PET study of patients at rest (Eidelberg et al., 1996). As a result, it appears that the recovery process following surgery may also involve the lateral premotor areas.

Conclusion A variety of related issues with movement control are frequently referred to as "bradykinesia." However, sluggish progress is always the primary drawback. Although secondary factors like muscle weakness, tremor, and rigidity may contribute, the primary deficit is caused by a lack of muscle force recruitment at the beginning of movement, according to the data examined here. As a consequence, the movements of patients miss their targets and eventually approach them in several smaller steps. The two distinctive elements of parkinsonian bradykinesia are (I) that patients underscale muscle power and (ii) that the shortfall is many times enhanced when outer signs (vision, sound) are given to direct the development. The previous has prompted the idea that bradykinesia is an issue of scaling engine yield properly to the undertaking as opposed to any characteristic constraint in engine execution. The latter is typically interpreted as a preference for medial rather than lateral motor cortical access for basal ganglia motor output. Medial cortical regions are more active when internal movements are generated, while lateral regions are more active when an external cue is given. In conclusion, the underscaling of movement commands in internally generated movements appears to be the primary cause of bradykinesia. This may indicate that the basal ganglia select and reinforce appropriate patterns of cortical activity during performance and preparation for a movement.

Other parts of the central nervous system can adapt to Parkinson's disease's deficit in the primary basal ganglia, as evidenced by recent imaging and EEG studies. As a result, the primary deficit and compensatory processes may come together in the clinical presentation of bradykinesia. We suggest that this interaction may be the cause of some aspects of bradykinesia, such as the inability to perform two tasks simultaneously and the progressive slowing of long movement sequences, as well as the long intervals between successive elements of a sequence. The argument can be developed further along this line. One of the new understandings of basal ganglia pathophysiology is that illness might make the basal ganglia yield loud. This noise may be removed or reduced in part by surgical interventions. The implication is that surgery improves function by allowing other structures to better compensate for the underlying deficit and by normalizing basal ganglia output.

Abstract: The disease known as cerebral malaria (CM) is caused by an infection with Plasmodium falciparum and has a high mortality rate. Seizures and neurocognitive deficits, which have a significant impact on a person's quality of life, are examples of post-CM sequelae that can last a lifetime for CM survivors. The neuropathogenesis that leads to these neurologic sequelae is unclear and understudied because the Plasmodium parasite does not enter the brain but instead lives inside erythrocytes and is confined to the lumen of the brain's vasculature. Postmortem CM pathology is interestingly different in different parts of the brain, like when haemorragic punctae appear in white matter versus gray matter. Exposure at a young age, genetics of the parasite and the host, parasite sequestration, and the extent of the host's inflammatory responses all increase the risk of CM. There have been several proposed adjunctive treatments for CM that have not been effective, but more are needed. The region-specific neuropathogenesis of CM that results in neurologic sequelae is intriguing, but research has not adequately addressed it. CM neurologic sequelae may be treated with effective adjunctive treatments if this gets more attention.

Background Female Anopheles mosquitoes infected with Plasmodium transmit malaria by biting. It continues to be one of the most prevalent diseases transmitted by vectors, resulting in high disease morbidity and mortality. Although there are a number of Plasmodium species that have the potential to cause disease, Plasmodium falciparum and Plasmodium vivax are the two main species that are responsible for the majority of human complications. P. vivax is more common in India and South East Asian countries. There were approximately 228 million cases of malaria and 405,000 deaths worldwide in 2016. 67% (272,000) of these deaths occurred in children under the age of 5.

The infection with P. falciparum can result in a number of complications, with cerebral malaria (CM) having some of the highest mortality rates. In addition, survivors of CM may suffer from post-CM sequelae that last a lifetime, particularly neurological deficits that impair quality of life. Serious jungle fever, because of P. falciparum disease, presents distinctively in youngsters than grown-ups, particularly with respect to the beginning of CM. Paediatric CM is linked to a higher rate of seizures and post-CM neurocognitive deficits, despite the fact that paediatric CM mortality is said to be lower than adult CM mortality. Different host responses of the cerebral vasculature in various brain regions to sequestration and the degree of inflammation may be the cause of these variations in the presentation of CM disease. The underlying immunopathophysiological mechanisms of pediatric P. falciparum malaria and its neurological sequelae in sub-Saharan Africa are the primary focus of this review.

Malaria is, from a genetic standpoint, the evolutionary driver resulting in genetic erythrocyte diseases such as sickle-cell, thalassaemia, and glucose-6-phosphate dehydrogenase deficiency, as more than one million children per year were dying from P. falciparum in Africa alone prior to the twenty-first century.

Host Genetic Susceptibility and Resistance

This is supported by the findings that, despite homozygote mortality, the HbS allele is prevalent in malaria-endemic regions and that distinct genetic mutations have emerged in diverse ethnic and geographic populations. Inflammatory factors and regulatory regions, such as Type 1 Interferon receptor variants in Malawi, IL17 in Nigeria, and IL4 and IL22 in populations in Mali, contribute to CM susceptibility. Additionally, intercellular adhesion molecular -1 (ICAM-1) Kilifi variants were implicated in CM in previous studies. NF polymorphisms were discovered in an Indian study and 15 genes were identified in a recent Kenyan study in Kilifi. Additionally, epidemiological studies demonstrated a correlation between age and prior exposure to epigenetic modifications and the outcomes of malaria infections. This is because it was recently discovered that severe malaria, including CM, increased the production of succinate and fumarate, metabolites of the citric acid cycle. These metabolites have the potential to modify epigenetic enzymes like DNA and histone demethylases. Invoking hyperresponsiveness of the Toll-like Receptors (TLR) ligand stimulation, recurrent parasite infections are increasingly being linked to epigenetic modifications that produce malaria-resistant phenotypes. In point of fact, children infected with Plasmodium in Kenya have been shown to exhibit these epigenetic modifications. Pediatric CM patients' concurrent infections, such as HIV, are regarded as distinct death risk factors. Studies of autopsies have shown that HIV-infected children who died from CM had twice as many intravascular monocytes and platelets. In addition, human CM brains with HIV co-infection showed an increased presence of T cells. T cell influx into the brain may be exacerbated in co-infected patients by HIV-associated immune dysregulation, likely amplifying CM pathological damage. Even though there are differences between regions, factors associated with strong host-immune responses appear to be crucial, as multiple host factors contribute to severe malaria susceptibility.

Clinical attributes

CM is the most extreme neurological difficulty of the contamination by P. falciparum and is a clinical disorder whose trademark is weakened cognizance, with unconsciousness being the most serious sign. A relapsing diurnal fever is one of the clinical signs of pediatric malaria, including CM. This fever is caused by the release of the parasite upon the rupture of Plasmodium infected red blood cells (PRBC) as a result of asexual replication and the release of cytokines. A diffuse CM encephalopathy, rapid progressive coma, seizures without regaining consciousness, or both can occur in acute infection patients. Occasionally, focal neurologic signs exist. Abnormal pupillary and corneal reflexes, a dysconjugate gaze, and irregular breathing patterns are common signs of brainstem dysfunction in children at the end of diseas. Long-term clinical follow-up assessments of paediatric CM survivors revealed an elevated persistence of neurological sequelae, including hemiplegia, ataxia, paresis, seizure disorders, language deficits, altered behavior, severe cerebral palsy, and cognitive impairments. Although some sequelae, such as cortical blindness, improve over time. These neurologic sequelae may prompt a hindered personal satisfaction and loss of inability changed life years. It is not clear what exact underlying factors contribute to the neuropathogenesis that results in poor neurological outcomes in children. Notwithstanding, dissection discoveries have determined that intravascular sequestration of Plasmodium-tainted red platelets is related with perivascular harm, including axonal injury, myelin misfortune and breakdown of the blood cerebrum boundary (BBB). It is unclear exactly how sequestration leads to BBB breakdown. Sequestration and soluble Plasmodium factors may have both direct and indirect effects on BBB integrity, which may be exacerbated by the cytokine storm and the influx of neurotoxic plasma factors like albumin. Postmortem pathology revealed various host vascular responses, but interestingly, sequestration reportedly occurs in the brain vasculature of pediatric African CM patients regardless of the region. Multiple haemorrhagic punctate lesions are more common in the white matter and corpus callosum, but they are not seen in the gray matter or basal ganglia. Postmortem pathology and magnetic resonance imaging (MRI) reveal that punctate white matter damage is also prevalent in adult P. falciparum CM. This suggests that different host responses may result from potential phenotypic heterogeneity in the local host vasculature that can attract differential PRBC sequestration.

Misdiagnosis is a possibility with the clinical World Health Organization (WHO) diagnostic criteria for CM (P. falciparum on blood smear, coma, and no other known cause of coma). A Malawian autopsy study found that 23% of clinically diagnosed CM cases actually had a completely different pathology based on these criteria. Because some children may already have neurocognitive issues, this has the potential to skew the results of post-CM cognitive studies. It has been demonstrated that fundoscopy and the diagnosis of retinopathy improve the specificity of the clinical diagnosis of CM, though adult retinopathy appears to be less specific. A constellation of ocular changes known as CM-retinopathy includes retinal whitening, retinal hemorrhages, vascular changes, papilledema, and elevated VCAM-1 expression.

Pathology

Pathology is a branch of medicine that studies abnormal conditions' structural and functional changes as well as their underlying causes. Early endeavors to concentrate on pathology were in many cases hindered by strict preclusions against post-mortem examinations, however these steadily loose during the late Medieval times, permitting dissections to decide the reason for death, the reason for pathology. The Italian Giovanni Battista Morgagni published the first systematic textbook of morbid anatomy in 1761, locating diseases within individual organs for the first time. This was the culmination of the resulting accumulation of anatomical information. It wasn't until the first half of the 19th century that clinical symptoms and pathological changes were found to be correlated.

A more scientific cellular theory took the place of the previous humoral theories of pathology; in 1858, Rudolf Virchow argued that the microscopic examination of diseased cells could reveal the nature of the condition. The final piece of information needed to comprehend numerous disease processes was provided by Louis Pasteur and Robert Koch's bacteriologic theory of disease, which was developed late in the 19th century.

By the end of the 19th century, pathology as a separate specialty had fairly established itself. The pathologist reports to and consults with the clinical physician, who directly cares for the patient, and does most of his work in the laboratory. The pathologist examines a variety of laboratory specimens, including surgically removed body parts, blood and other body fluids, urine, feces, and other exudates, and so on. Through the process of autopsy, pathology practice also includes reconstructing the final chapter of a deceased person's physical life, which provides valuable information about disease processes that would otherwise be unavailable. Subspecialists collaborate whenever conditions permit because the knowledge required for proper general pathology practice cannot be achieved by a single individual. Neuropathology, pediatric pathology, general surgical pathology, dermatopathology, and forensic pathology are among the laboratory subspecialties that pathologists work in.

The pathologist now has access to a plethora of chemical stains, finer definition of subcellular structures with the electron microscope, easier access to internal organs for biopsy with the use of glass fiber-optic instruments, and microbial cultures for the purpose of identifying infectious diseases.

Prior to admission to pathology postgraduate programs, formal medical education with an M.D. degree or its equivalent is required in many Western nations. Five years of postgraduate education and training are required for board certification as a pathologist.

White nose syndrome is a disease that affects hibernating bats in North America. It is brought on by the growth of a white fungus called Pseudogymnoascus destructans in the skin of the nose, ears, and wings. White nose syndrome is the first known epizootic (epidemic) disease that has been linked to a high mortality rate in bats. In the first six years following its discovery in February 2006 at Howe Caverns near Albany, New York, biologists estimated that between 5.7 and 6.7 million bats died from white nose syndrome, with some colonies experiencing declines of more than 90%.

White nose syndrome's emergence and spread were first documented in 2007, when as many as 11,000 bats with symptoms of a fungal infection perished in caves near Albany. The disease then spread to New England and was discovered in caves in the

Appalachian Mountains, including ones in Canada, New Brunswick, and as far south as Tennessee, South Carolina, and Georgia in the United States. It was also found in Nova Scotia, Ontario, and Quebec, as well as far west as Wisconsin, Missouri, and Arkansas in the United States.

In 2008 researchers effectively separated and refined the organism and the next year distinguished it as another species, Geomyces destructans. The newly discovered organism was reclassified and renamed as a result of the organism's subsequent genetic evaluation and comparisons with closely related fungi, which revealed a high degree of similarity to fungi in the genus Pseudogymnoascus. However, its origin remained a mystery. P. destructans was found in European bats, which are less likely to die from infection, suggesting that it was present in Europe before North America. Genetic variations in P. destructans isolates taken from bats in Europe and North America provided evidence to support this hypothesis. P. destructans isolates from European bats showed a lot of genetic variation depending on where they were found, indicating that the species has been around for a long time in Europe. In contrast, the genetic diversity of the isolates from North American bats was relatively low, indicating that the fungus only entered North America once and then spread from there. Consequently, it is conceivable that P. destructans was acquainted with North America from Europe, reasonable having been helped by people, since bats don't move between the two landmasses.

P. destructans is psychrophilic, which means that it likes cold. It grows best at temperatures between 4 and 15 °C (39.2 and 59 °F) and 90% or higher humidity, which is about the same range as the temperature and humidity found in bat hibernacula. Bats appear to be most susceptible to infection during torpor and hibernation because they are close to the pathogen and have a significantly slowed immune system and metabolism. Additionally, it is believed that bats are infected with P. destructans when they come into contact with the fungus in cave environments, although the exact transmission method is unknown. The fungus can also be passed between bats through physical contact, and it might even be passed between bats and other animals, including humans. Such contagiousness proposes that the organism can be spread quickly to new regions through bats' day to day and occasional developments, including significant distance relocation.

Characteristics that contribute to disease P. destructans stands out from other fungal skin pathogens due to its capacity to enter connective tissue and subcutaneous tissues, including superficial skin layers. The wing membrane is where fungal hyphae (filaments) penetrate the thin cutaneous layers to produce visible erosions (small cuplike lesions) that house a significant fungal biomass, including conidia (asexual spores). This is the most obvious sign of infection. The fungus may spread beneath the abrasions into the specialized connective tissues of the wing, where it can cause significant functional damage that compromises the wing's elasticity, tensile strength, and tone. It may also affect the flow of blood and gas exchange between the lungs across the membrane of the wing.

Bats are repeatedly awoken from hibernation by fungal invasion through the skin, which appears to cause physiological changes that disrupt thermoregulation and force them to burn extra energy to stay warm. Bats with severely damaged wings and depleted fat stores eventually perish. While certain setbacks tumble to the floor of their hibernacula, others have been tracked down actually gripping to buckle walls. In other instances, affected bats may exhibit unusual behavior, such as leaving their hibernacula in the middle of the winter in search of food and water, often succumbing to starvation, dehydration, or exposure to the cold. Even if affected bats make it through the winter, they might not fly as well, which could affect how well they can forage and reproduce. Immune reconstitution inflammatory syndrome is a condition in which the immune system responds to the remaining infection with an overwhelming inflammatory response that significantly damages the wing tissues and results in death for some infected survivors.

Future effects and the board

A portion of the primary species in North America where white nose condition was identified incorporated the little earthy colored bat (Myotis lucifugus), the imperiled Indiana bat (M. sodalis), and the large earthy colored bat (Eptesicus fuscus). Since then, the disease has been found in a number of other endangered species. However, due to the fact that more than 20 bat species inhabit the contiguous United States and Canada and hibernate, it is likely that they are susceptible to white nose syndrome. For instance, the northern long-eared bat (M. septentrionalis) experienced significant declines, which resulted in its designation as a threatened species under the Endangered Species Act of the United States. Additionally, due to the fact that many North American bats are insectivorous, their extinction could result in an increase in the number of insects, which could have an effect on the health of forests, agriculture, and human health.

Researchers have been attempting to recognize ways of outmaneuvering deal with the spread of P. destructans. Nonetheless, PC recreated separating models and examinations of other conceivable administration approaches have uncovered the difficulties confronting control endeavors. For instance, the fact that P. destructans was found in cave sediments suggests that the pathogen has a reservoir in the environment. This would make it impossible to control the disease by killing infected bats. A DNA test that was sensitive enough to detect P. destructans in soil samples from bat hibernacula and wing skin samples from live bats was reported by scientists in 2013. The strategy was undeniably more delicate than recently utilized tests and was supposed to facilitate testing of bats and cavern substrates for the growth, empowering early discovery and further developed control of the illness.

Karl, Aristocrat Von Rokitansky:

Austrian pathologist

Karl, aristocrat von Rokitansky, (conceived Feb. 19, 1804, Königgrätz, Austria — kicked the bucket July 23, 1878, Vienna), Austrian pathologist whose undertakings to lay out an efficient image of the wiped out living being from almost 100,000 post-mortem examinations — 30,000 of which he, at the end of the day, performed — assisted make the investigation of obsessive life structures a foundation of present day clinical practice and laid out the New Vienna With tutoring as a world clinical focus during the last 50% of the nineteenth hundred years.

He was a professor of pathological anatomy at the Vienna General Hospital from 1844 to 1974. He encouraged the Bohemian student Ignaz Semmelweis, who later became a martyr for the cause of antiseptic medical practice, to study medicine in 1846 and helped him clean Europe's maternity wards to get rid of childbed fever.

First to distinguish microorganisms in quite a while of threatening endocarditis, a frequently quickly deadly irritation of the layer covering the internal walls of the heart, Rokitansky made the reason for a separation of lobar pneumonia (starting in the lower curve of the lung) and lobular pneumonia, or bronchopneumonia (beginning in the better developments of the extended bronchial tree). He made a key investigation of intense yellow decay of the liver (presently known as

Rokitansky's sickness; 1843), first described spondylolisthesis, the forward displacement of one vertebra over another, and established the micropathology of pulmonary emphysema, a condition of the lung characterized by enlarged air spaces separated from the terminals of the bronchial tree (1839).

His three-volume Pathological Anatomie Handbook 1842–46; Treatise of Pathological Anatomy, published between 1849 and 1852), marked the advancement of the field to the level of a well-established science.

Printed in the USA
CPSIA information can be obtained
at www.ICGtesting.com
LVHW020737161124
796811LV00014B/862